ANTI-INFLAMMATORY VEGAN DIET FOR BEGINNERS

How to lose weight in 28 days with vegan recipes. The diet cookbook that in 4 weeks will allow you to restore your immune system and heal inflammation

ERIKA MELANDRI

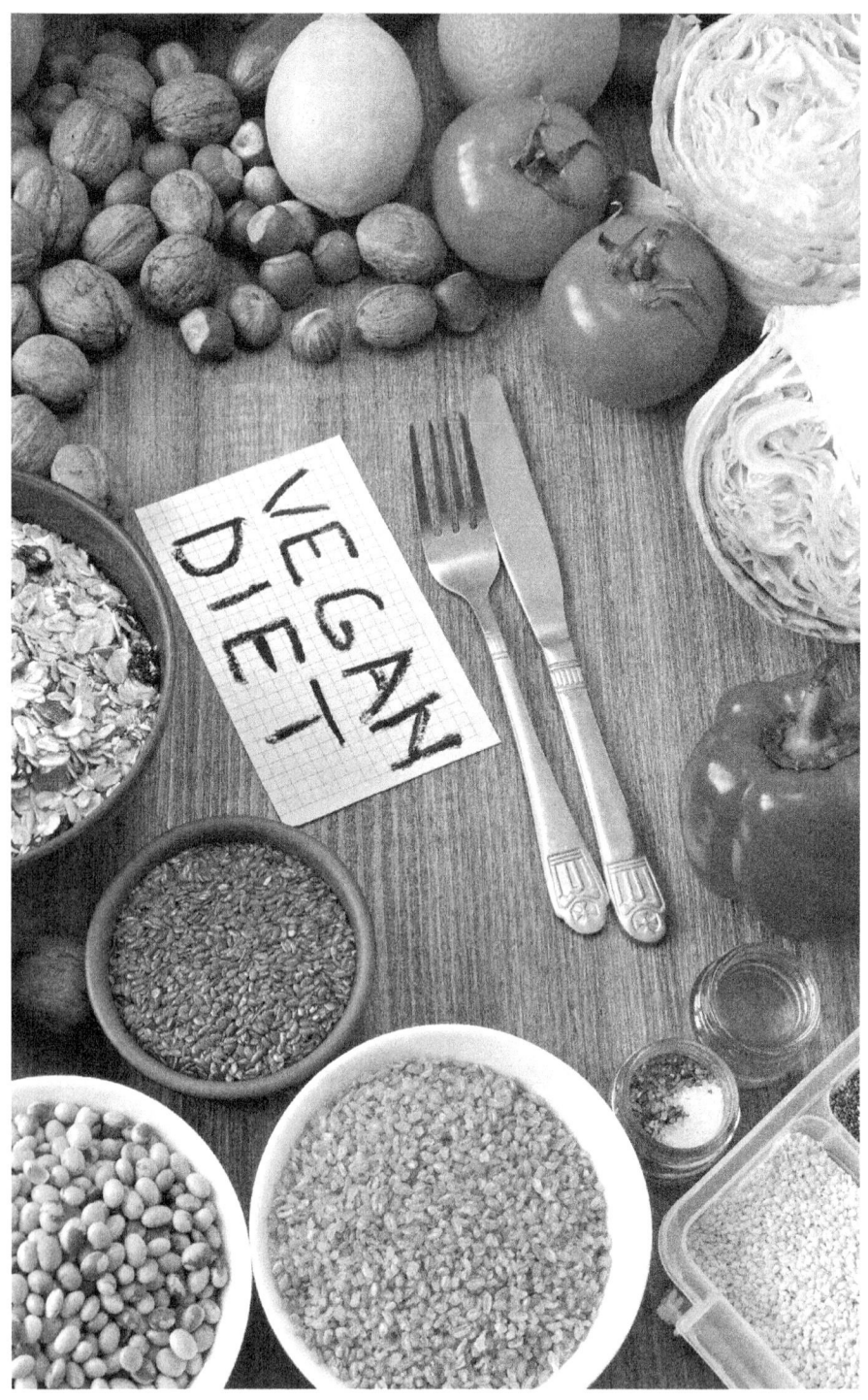

Contents

INTRODUCTION 10
HOW TO APPLY THE EASY 28-DAY METHOD 19
BREAKFAST VEGAN 23
SCRAMBLED TOFU 26
SEITAN CHORIZO 29
MIGAS 32
RUSTIC TEMPEH SAUSAGES 35
COFFEE CAKE 38
HASH BROWNS 42
PANCAKES 45
CREPES 48
WAFFLES 52
GOOD MORNING MUFFINS 55
APPETIZER AND SNACKS 59
PREVIEW 60
TUSCAN WHITE BEAN SPREAD 61
BLACK BEAN DIP 64
CURRIED LENTILS DIP 67
GUACAMOLE 70
SKORDALIA 73
CAPONATA 76
TOSTONES 80

SWEET POTATO FALAFEL	83
VEGAN CHILI RELLENOS	86
SOUP PASTA AND BREADS	90
VEGETABLE STOCK	93
GREEN VEGETABLE BROTH	96
MISO SOUP	99
ONION SOUP	102
LENTIL AND SPINACH SOUP	105
ORECCHIETTE WITH BUTTERNUT SQUASH	108
AVOCADO SOUP	112
FARFALLE WITH SUN DRIED TOMATOES AND PORTOBELLO	115
MACARONI AND CHEESE	118
COUSCOUS WITH RAISINS AND PINE NUTS	121
POTATO AND ROSEMARY PIZZA	124
WHITE PIZZA WITH TOFU BOURSIN	127
RUSTIC PIE	130
VEGETABLE AND SOY FOODS	135
ARTICHOKE AND ARUGULA SALAD	138
GRILLED ASPARAGUS AND LEEKS WITH ALMONDS	141
ROASTED BROCCOLI	144
TUNISIAN CARROT SALAD	147
CAULIFLOWER WITH CAPERS	150
EGGPLANT ROLLATINI	153
GREEN BEANS WITH ALMONDS AND MUSTARD	156

GLAZED TOFU	159
AFGHAN SPINACH AND TOFU	162
TOFU CURRY IN PUMPKIN	165
EDAMAME WITH HIJIKI AND BROWN RICE	169
TEMPEH IN TOMATO SAUCE	172
CONDIMENTS AND SAUCE SALADS AND DRESSING	176
TOFU MAYONNAISE	179
COOKING KETCHUP	182
HOT MUSTARD	185
OLIVE DRESSING	188
GREEN TOMATO SEASONING	191
OKRA PICKLES	194
MUSHROOM PESTO	197
DESSERTS AND BEVERAGE	201
YELLOW CAKE	203
THICK CHOCOLATE GANACHE	206
LINZER COOKIE SQUARES	209
MANGO CREAM PIE	212
EASY PEACH CRISP	215
SOFT-SERVE ICE CREAM	218
BANANA MILK	221
CREAMY ORANGE SMOOTHIE	224
STRAWBERRY AND BASIL LEMONADE	227
FINAL CONCLUSIONS	232

© Copyright 2022 by Erika Melandri - All rights reserved.

The following Book is reproduced below with the goal of providing information that is as accurate and reliable as possible. Regardless, purchasing this Book can be seen as consent to the fact that both the publisher and the author of this book are in no way experts on the topics discussed within and that any recommendations or suggestions that are made herein are for entertainment purposes only. Professionals should be consulted as needed prior to undertaking any of the action endorsed herein.

This declaration is deemed fair and valid by both the American Bar Association and the Committee of Publishers Association and is legally binding throughout the United States.

Furthermore, the transmission, duplication, or reproduction of any of the following work including specific information will be considered an illegal act irrespective of if it is done electronically or in print. This extends to creating a secondary or tertiary copy of the work or a recorded copy and is only allowed with the express written consent from the Publisher. All additional right reserved.

The information in the following pages is broadly considered a truthful and accurate account of facts and as such, any inattention, use, or misuse of the information in question by the reader will render any resulting actions solely under their purview. There are no scenarios in which the publisher or the original author of this work can be in any fashion deemed liable for any hardship or damages that may befall them after undertaking information described herein.

Additionally, the information in the following pages is intended only for informational purposes and should thus be thought of as universal. As befitting its nature, it is presented without assurance regarding its prolonged validity or interim quality. Trademarks that are mentioned are done without written consent and can in no way be considered an endorsement from the trademark holder.

INTRODUCTION

The vegan diet is a dietary regimen that provides for the exclusion of all foods of animal origin and, consequently, provides for the intake of plant foods only.
All people who follow a vegan diet, besides not eating foods of animal origin, do not even consume their products and their derivatives such as milk and derivatives, eggs and honey precisely because it is assumed that animals have been exploited to obtain them. Besides the food aspect, therefore, this choice also involves ethical aspects of respect for animals.
The vegan diet is very suitable to detoxify the body from toxins that come from foods of animal origin, mainly from red meat and dairy products.
Foods that, especially if taken frequently and in large quantities, can lead to obstruction of the bloodstream and consequent inflammation, affecting the intestine but not only, with manifestations such as lack of physical energy, anemia, migraine, obesity, osteoporosis, up to cancer.
Moreover, the digestion of these foods leads to the formation of large amounts of free radicals, chemical molecules very reactive and harmful to tissues.
Conversely, the intake of large quantities of fruits and vegetables has a beneficial antioxidant action.

With a targeted selection of vegan foods and good planning, it is possible without having deficiencies of essential nutrients. If you eat vegan food, you should especially have an adequate intake of nutrients such as protein, omega-3 fatty acids, vitamin B2, calcium, iron, iodine, zinc and selenium through appropriate foods. Because vitamin B12 cannot be produced by plants and animal foods containing vitamin B12 cannot be consumed by vegans, the DGE recommends the use of fortified foods or supplements with appropriate preparations, such as chlorella. Find out more about foods with vitamin B12 for vegans!

Daily vitamin D requirements can be largely covered by direct sunlight through skin self-synthesis. Typically, 15-30 minutes in the sun is enough to produce sufficient vitamin D. Since very few plant foods contain significant amounts of fat-soluble vitamins, it may be helpful to use a vitamin D supplement - for example in the form of vitamin D capsules. Combining plant foods with foods or juices containing vitamin C can lead to improved iron intake, as vitamin C increases iron absorption.

Find out how to cover your protein needs naturally with the best vegan protein sources, how you can lose weight, and how to eradicate pesky inflammation generated by poor nutrition through my recipes and method I've called 28 Days and Back Happy.

VEGAN HISTORY

It is 1944 when the two members of the Vegetarian Society, Donald Watson, and Elsie Shrigley, gather in one group the six vegetarians who had decided not to consume any product of animal origin, give life to the Vegan Society.

On this very day, therefore, the term Vegan appears for the first time, coined by Watson as a contraction of Vegetarian. A word that is not accidental and that encloses the thought of its founder: according to Watson, in fact, the vegan philosophy had to be the "beginning and end of vegetarianism."

And it is in memory of this day that every year, on November 1, vegans worldwide celebrate World Vegan Day.

THE PRINCIPLES OF VEGAN PHILOSOPHY

Contrary to what one might believe, the vegan philosophy is not based on an aversion to the killing of animals but on the refusal to adhere to a lifestyle based on the intensive and systematic exploitation of all forms of life.

In line with a non-violent vision of life and with the principles of anti-speciesist thought, therefore, the vegan philosophy includes the detachment from activities in which man exercises absolute power over the lives of other animals (such as animal breeding for human consumption, experimentation on animals, or hunting).

Although there are no fixed criteria for all vegans, those who decide to adopt a lifestyle of this type must reject not only foods of animal origin but also a whole range of everyday products such as cosmetics, clothing, or cleaning products.

TYPES OF COOKING IN THE VEGAN DIETS

Talking about Vegan Nutrition also means considering the different methods used for cooking food.

Besides the most common types of cooking, such as boiling, steaming, grilling, or baking, there are also some rather particular ones that are worth mentioning:

Nischimè: cooking on a very low flame with water and without the use of oil. Vegetables are also cut into pieces of 2-3 centimeters and arranged in layers, from the hardest to the softest.

Stir-frying: vegetables are stir-fried in a pan in three different ways: with oil, with water, without oil, or water.

Tempura: it is the typical Japanese frying that foresees the immersion of food in a batter of water and flour before being fried in oil.

In Vegan Nutrition, it is used for cooking foods such as seitan, tofu, seaweeds, and edible flowers.

ABOUT ME

Hi, my name is Erika Melandri, and I am a nutritionist with a great passion for cooking...

I am of Italian Origin so you can understand very well that when we talk about eating, we are talking about serious things...

Before graduating, I attended for 2 years the Hotel School, the most renowned in my city, obviously choosing the kitchen as the hotel industry...

I know very well all the international cuisines, and the degree has allowed me to deepen all the aspects of diets and weight loss programs of all kinds ...

I also have a great passion for writing, and after receiving major awards as a chef and as a dietitian-nutritionist, I decided to write my works and my methods based on the simplicity of use that, if followed precisely, leads to certain results in terms of both weight loss and above all bring back and maintain the most important metabolic values at a normal level...

On this my author page, you will find books on Italian and international cuisine, but above all, dietary books with my method Easy 28 days and back in shape and happy.

Remember that eating healthy associated with a little physical activity is the secret to maintaining youth, health, and well-being, both physical and mental.

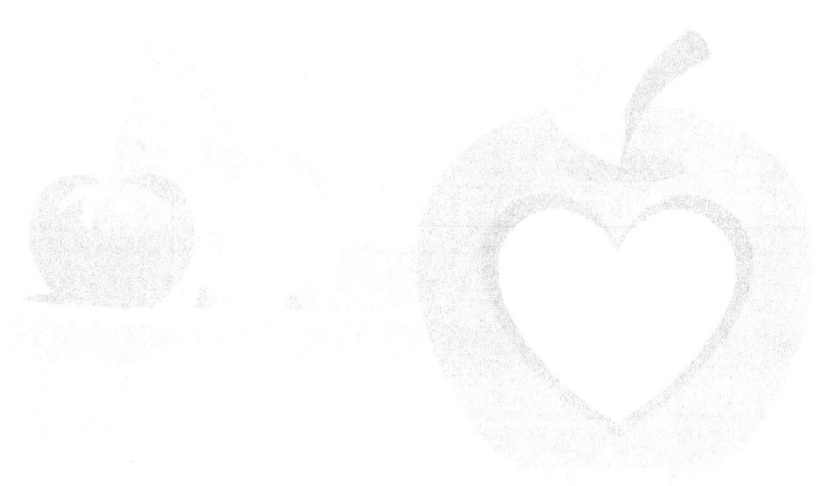

HOW TO APPLY THE EASY 28-DAY METHOD

I have prepared for you a system that I called 28 days to bet in 4 steps....

You can choose yourself 1 recipe among the many you will find in this recipe book.
The table that you will find on the next page will explain in a simple way how to use it.

The system involves eating a course of your choice three times a day, I guarantee you won't feel hungry, and you won't have to sacrifice too much.

Want to bet that I can get you to lose about 7-10 pounds in 28 days?

Eat healthy and get back into physical shape.

Now I'll explain specifically the easy method.

In the table below I will explain a very precise program that is divided into 4 weeks where each week you will have to follow a food line choosing at will from the 6 main meals that I have included in this book.

Let's see them together:

VEGAN BREAKFAST, APPETIZER AND SNACKS, SOUP PASTA AND BREAD, PLANT FOODS AND SOY, SALAD DRESSINGS AND DRESSING, DESSERTS AND DRINKS.

Each meal contains many recipes to have a variety that allows you to choose the one that best suits your taste.

You will need to choose a different one by following the table on the next page.

Example: Monday choose a recipe for breakfast, 1 recipe for lunch and 1 recipe for dinner.

Tuesday the same thing, choose another recipe to taste and so on ... you can choose as many recipes as you want, the important thing is to follow the table that will be presented on the next page, simple, fast and that will have an immediate impact in the first week.

Want to bet?

Now let's get to work, it's time to start....

Week	Mon	Tue	Wed	Thu	Fri	Sat	Sun
1°	**Breakfast** Choose a recipe among many **Lunch** Soup **Dinner** Vegetable	**Breakfast** Choose a recipe among many **Lunch** Breads **Dinner** Beans and Grain	**Breakfast** choose a recipe among many **Lunch** Snack **Dinner** Soy food	**Breakfast** choose a recipe among many **Lunch** Soup **Dinner** Snack	**Breakfast** choose a recipe among many **Lunch** Vegetable+ Condiments **Dinner** Pizza	**Breakfast** choose a recipe among many **Lunch** Soup and Snack+Dessert **Dinner** Vegetable Soy food	**Breakfast** choose a recipe among many **Lunch** Breads+ Dessert **Dinner** Beans and Grain
2°	**Breakfast** Choose a recipe among many **Lunch** Breads **Dinner** Beans and Grain	**Breakfast** Choose a recipe among many **Lunch** Soup or Pasta **Dinner** Vegetable +Sauce	**Breakfast** choose a recipe among many **Lunch** Soup **Dinner** Snack	**Breakfast** choose a recipe among many **Lunch** Snack **Dinner** Soy food	**Breakfast** Choose a recipe among many **Lunch** Soup or Pizza **Dinner** Vegetable	**Breakfast** choose a recipe among many **Lunch** Vegetable **Dinner** Pizza+ Dessert	**Breakfast** choose a recipe among many **Lunch** Soup and Snack+Dessert **Dinner** Vegetable Soy food
3°	**Breakfast** Choose a recipe among many **Lunch** Soup or Pasta **Dinner** Vegetable	**Breakfast** choose a recipe among many **Lunch** Snack **Dinner** Soy food	**Breakfast** Choose a recipe among many **Lunch** Breads **Dinner** Beans and Grain	**Breakfast** choose a recipe among many **Lunch** Soup **Dinner** Snack+ Appetizer	**Breakfast** choose a recipe among many **Lunch** Snack **Dinner** Soy food	**Breakfast** choose a recipe among many **Lunch** Breads+ Dessert **Dinner** Beans and Grain	**Breakfast** choose a recipe among many **Lunch** Soup and Snack+Dessert **Dinner** Vegetable Soy food
4°	**Breakfast** choose a recipe among many **Lunch** Vegetable+ Sauce **Dinner** Pizza	**Breakfast** Choose a recipe among many **Lunch** Soup **Dinner** Vegetable+ Souce	**Breakfast** choose a recipe among many **Lunch** Snack **Dinner** Soy food	**Breakfast** choose a recipe among many **Lunch** Soup or Pasta **Dinner** Snack	**Breakfast** Choose a recipe among many **Lunch** Soup **Dinner** Vegetable	**Breakfast** choose a recipe among many **Lunch** Breads+ Dessert **Dinner** Beans and Grain	**Breakfast** choose a recipe among many **Lunch** Soup and Snack+Dessert **Dinner** Vegetable Soy food

TABLE

Now it's time to reveal my recipes enjoy them

BREAKFAST VEGAN

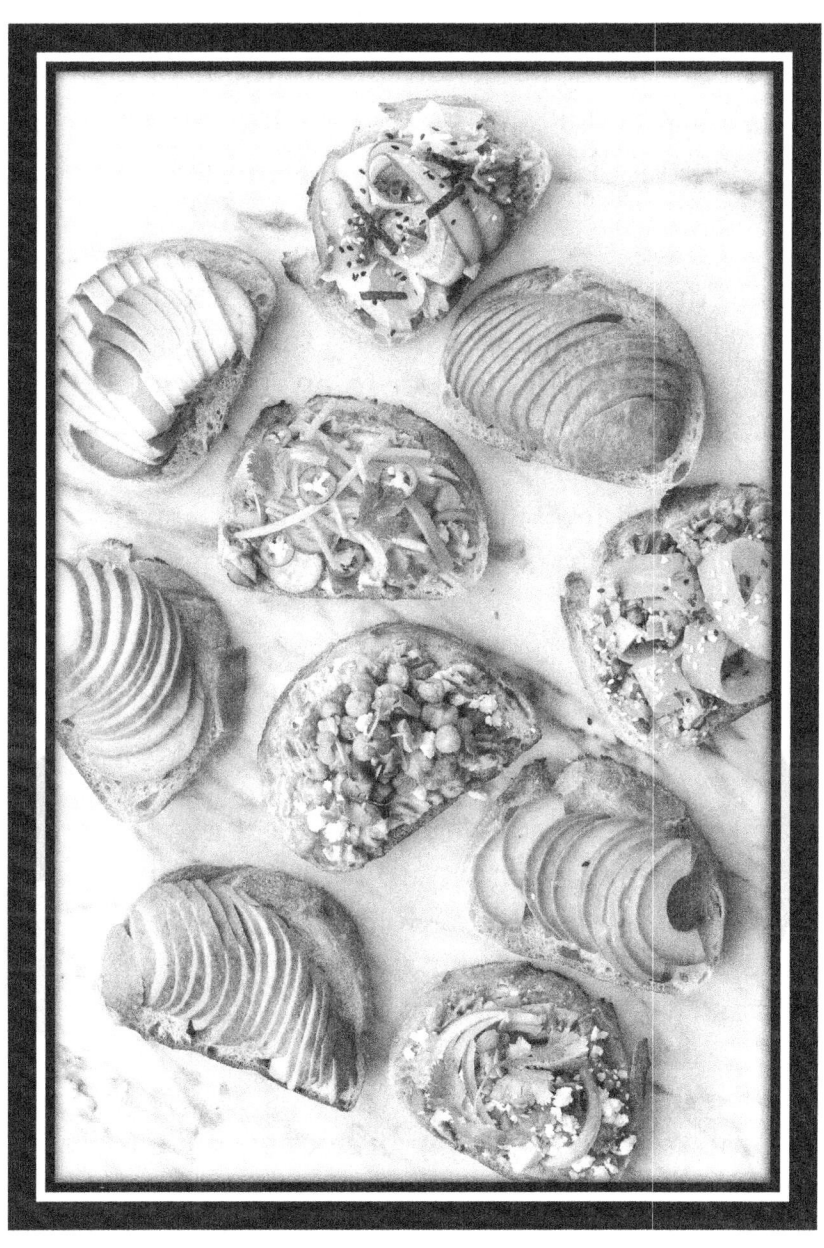

PREVIEW

A vegan breakfast does not contain foods of animal origin, but it should still be able to provide all the fundamental nutrients needed to maintain nutritional balance.

Recipes for a good vegan breakfast are both sweet, therefore pertinent, for example, to an Italian breakfast, and savory, closer to an American breakfast.

The most used foods in vegan breakfast can be divided in two big macro groups: Solid foods, Liquid foods.

I will try to give you various alternatives to solve this little obstacle.

To improve the palatability of the diet, it is therefore necessary to add creativity to the recipes, from breakfast to dinner. In the following paragraph, I will propose some food combinations to vary our "vegan breakfast" to the maximum.

Below you will find several examples of vegan recipes, tasty and relevant to vegan breakfast, have fun and choose a different recipe for each day to your liking.

SCRAMBLED TOFU

In most grocery stores, you can find pre-packaged mixes for processing tofu, but it's very easy to make on your own as well. Turmeric is used more for color than for flavor. If you are you are too tired in the morning to handle a knife, substitute ½ teaspoon of onion powder and ¼ teaspoon of garlic powder for the vegetables.

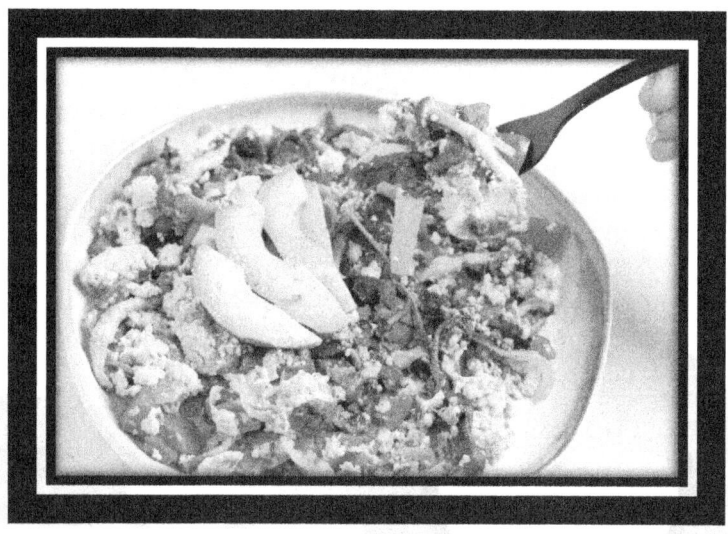

Ingredients:
Servings:2

- 2 teaspoons oil
- 2 teaspoons soy sauce
- 1 small onion, diced
- 1 teaspoon minced garlic
- 1 green bell pepper
- 8 ounces of tofu

- 1 tablespoon nutritional yeast
- ¼ teaspoon ground turmeric

Description:

Sauté onion in a skillet with hot oil, add garlic and green pepper until the onion is soft. Crumble the tofu well into the vegetables. Add the yeast, turmeric, and soy sauce. Mix thoroughly and heat through.

Nutrition values:
Calories: 108,Fat: 4.6 g,Cholesterol: 0 mg,Protein: 10 g,Carbohydrates: 9.2 g,Sugar: 3.5 g,Fiber: 4.2 g,Calcium: 67 mg

SEITAN CHORIZO

This spicy Spanish sausage can be served for breakfast or used in casseroles like Millet Paella. The flax seeds in this recipe help hold the link together and give it a very realistic texture, but the recipe works well without them.

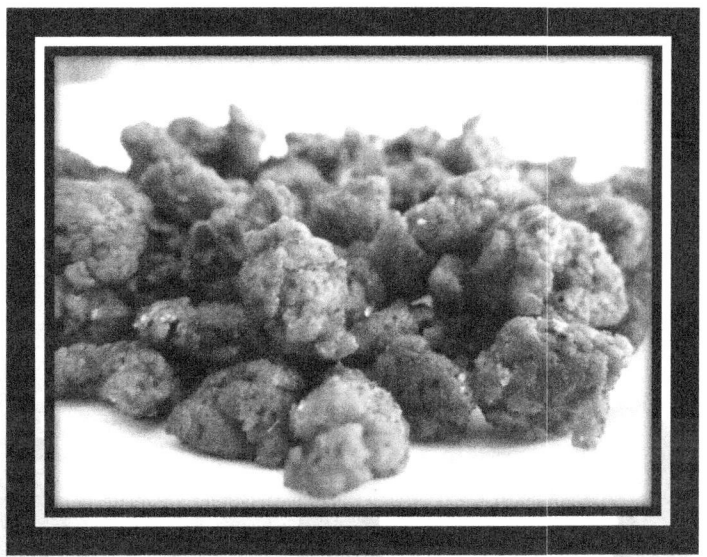

Ingredients:
Servings:4

- 1 tablespoon flaxseed
- ½ teaspoon fennel seeds
- ¼ teaspoon dried oregano
- 1 pound seitan, finely chopped
- 1 cup dry red wine
- 1 tablespoon soy sauce
- 2 tablespoons canola oil

- ½ cup finely diced yellow onion
- 2 teaspoons minced garlic
- 1 teaspoon cayenne
- 1 teaspoon ground cumin
- 2 teaspoons paprika, preferably smoked paprika
- 2 teaspoons of black pepper

Description:

In a small food processor, grind flax seeds with ¼ cup of water.
Pour into a small bowl and cover.
In a large nonstick skillet, lightly heat the oil over medium heat. Sauté the onion, garlic and dry spices until the onion is soft and a strong aroma rises from the pan. Add the seitan and heat through. Add 1 cup of red wine and soy sauce to the skillet and cook until the mixture is dry. Remove the skillet from the heat. Stir in flax seeds left aside.
Adjust seasonings.
When the mixture has cooled, you can handle it well—shape sausage into patties or links. Cook the formed sausages in a clean skillet over medium heat with more canola oil until well browned, about 5-7 minutes on each side. The sausages can be cooked and frozen for later use.

Nutrition values:
Calories: 96,Fat: 4 g,Cholesterol: 0 mg,Protein: 10 g,Carbohydrates: 6.2 g,Sugar: 3.5 g,Fiber: 4.2 g,Calcium: 32 mg

MIGAS

Migas in Spanish means tortilla strips or strips that are scrambled together with whatever vegetables you have in your refrigerator. Despite its simple name, this is a dish with unique flavors because of the variety of ingredients. For a quick breakfast, roll the Migas in a whole wheat tortilla and serve to taste with a light sauce.

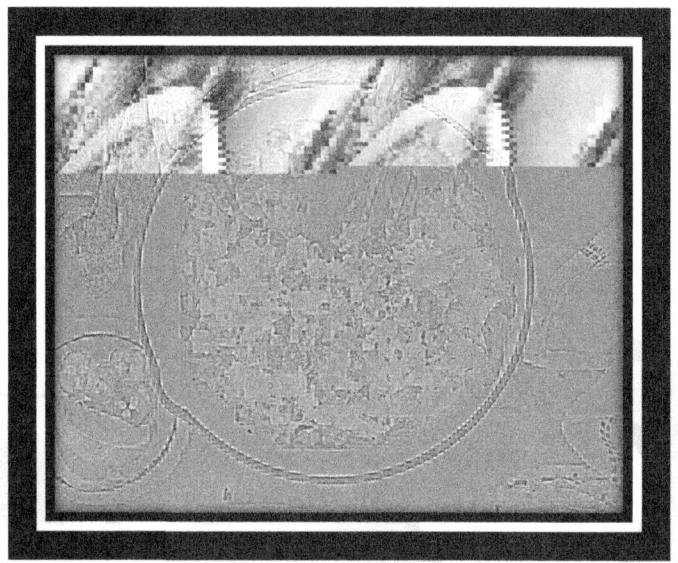

Ingredients:
Servings: 2

- 2 teaspoons of oil
- 1 pound of tofu
- 1 medium onion, diced
- 2 teaspoons minced garlic
- 1 medium red bell pepper, diced

- 1 small jalapeño, chopped
- 1 medium green bell pepper, diced
- 1 teaspoon turmeric
- ¼ teaspoon ground cumin
- 1 tablespoon nutritional yeast
- 1 medium tomato, diced
- 2 tablespoons chopped fresh cilantro
- 1 tablespoon soy sauce
- 2 corn tortillas

Description:

Cut the tortillas into strips.
Put heat extra virgin olive oil in a medium-sized frying pan. Saute the onion with the garlic and peppers until the onion is soft. Stir and add turmeric and cumin to the vegetables. Crumble the tofu into the vegetables. Add the yeast, tomato, cilantro, and soy sauce and mix well. Add the tortillas cut into strips and heat through.

Nutrition values:
334 calories; protein 14.1g; carbohydrates 42g; dietary fiber 7.5g; sugars 5.2g; fat 14.4g; saturated fat 1.7g

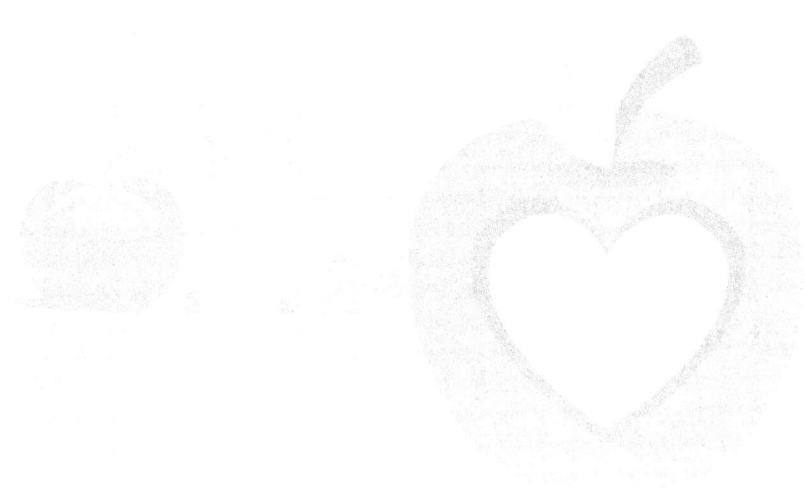

RUSTIC TEMPEH SAUSAGES

Tempeh is a fermented soybeans, delicious to cook in so many ways including escalope!

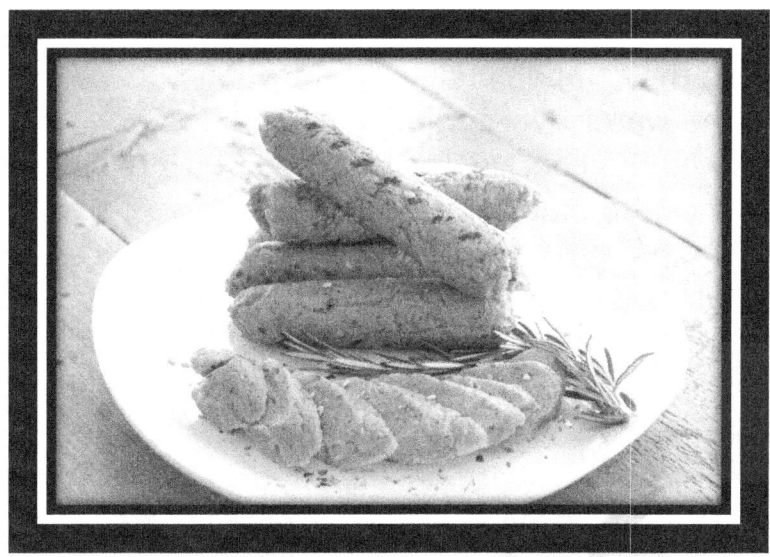

Ingredients:
Servings:4

- Two packages of tempeh, cut into cubes
- Canola oil for frying
- ¼ teaspoon pepper
- ½ cup whole wheat flour
- ½ teaspoon dried thyme
- 1½ teaspoons dried sage
- ¼ teaspoon dried savory
- ½ teaspoon red pepper flakes
- 1 tablespoon soy sauce
- ¼ cup olive oil

Description:

Steam the tempeh in boiling water for 15 minutes. Alternatively, you can microwave the tempeh, cover with microwave-safe plastic wrap for 1 to 2 minutes, or place the tempeh cubes in a bowl and pour 2 cups of boiling water over them.

Cover well the container with a clean dish towel and let sit for 15 minutes. Drain.

Crumble the tempeh well and add the dry spices and mix well. Add the flour, soy sauce, and oil and mix well. Let the sausage rest for 10 to 15 minutes. With moistened hands, form about eight meatballs from the mixture. Place the resulting patties (about 8) on a baking sheet lined with baking paper. Chill for 1 hour. Cook the meatballs in a clean medium-sized skillet over medium heat with canola oil until well browned, about 5 minutes on each side.

The sausages can be cooked and frozen, and used later.

Nutrition values:

Calories: 264, Carbs: 49 g, Fat: 3 g, Protein: 11 g, Sodium: 568 mg

COFFEE CAKE

Coffee Cake is simple to prepare yet delicious cake typical of American breakfast.
The Coffee Cake lends itself to various interpretations and reworkings, both in form and taste. Here we have the vegan version that will amaze you ... You can make it square or make single small portions by baking it in a muffin tin. You can enrich it with seasonal fruit or stuff it with a few spoonfuls of jam in the dough. The crumble, instead, can be enriched with toasted almonds.

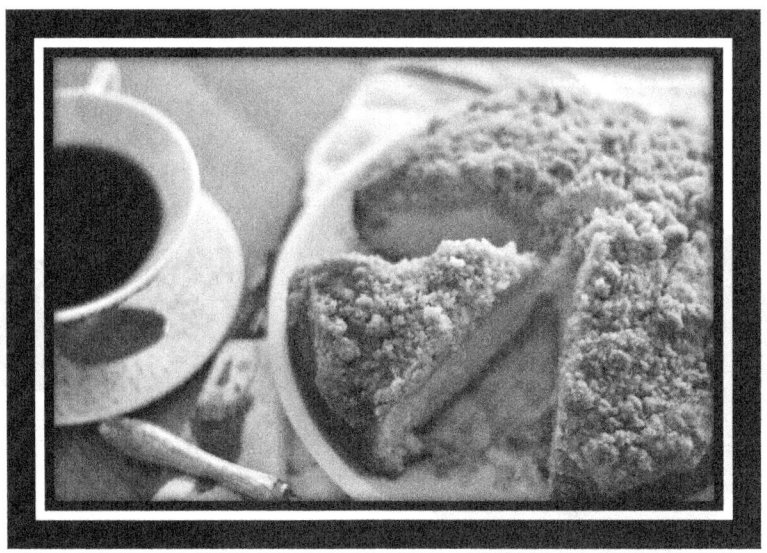

Ingredients:
Servings:4

- 1/2 cup brown sugar
- 1/2 cup whole wheat flour
- ½ teaspoon ground cinnamon

- 1 cup chopped nuts (optional)
- 2 tablespoons canola oil
- 1 cup all-purpose flour
- 1 cup sugar
- ¾ teaspoon baking soda
- ½ teaspoon ground cinnamon
- ¼ teaspoon ground nutmeg
- ¼ teaspoon salt
- 1 cup vegan sour cream or 6 ounces silken tofu blended with 1 tablespoon lemon juice and 1 tablespoon
- oil
- 2 teaspoons vanilla extract

Description:

Mix the brown sugar, whole wheat flour, cinnamon, and nuts. Add the oil and blend. If the mixture is too crumbly to make a good streusel, add 1 tablespoon of water and blend until it resembles coarse crumbs. Grease an 8-inch square baking dish. Preheat the oven to 350°.

Mix the all-purpose flour, sugar, baking soda, cinnamon, nutmeg, and salt in a medium bowl. Stir in the sour cream and vanilla. Stir just until the mixture is blended. Pour the batter into the prepared pan. Top evenly with the streusel mixture—Bake for 25 to 30 minutes.

Nutritional values:
energy 1582 kJ / 378 kcal, fat 15 g, saturated fat 4.3 g, carbohydrates 60 g, sugar 39 g, protein 3.7 g, salt 0.9 g.

HASH BROWNS

There are endless variations in the preparation of this breakfast. I for one, prefer slicing the potatoes rather than grating them, but either method works. The real trick is not to rush but let the onions caramelize, and the potatoes get crispy before flipping. E use a metal or rubber spatula if you're using a nonstick pan(I recommend it).

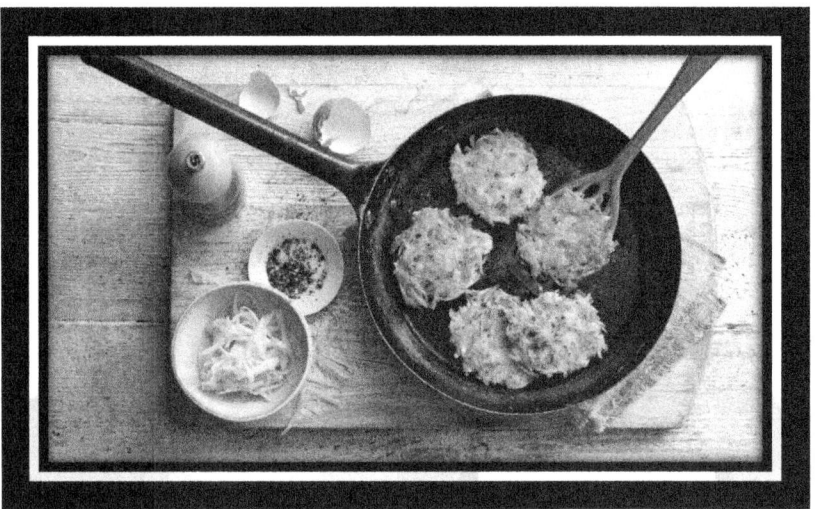

Ingredients:
Servings:4

- 1 1/2 pounds potatoes
- 1 medium onion
- 3 garlic cloves, peeled
- Oil
- Salt and freshly ground black pepper

Description:

Take a pot with 2 liters of cold water and put it on the fire, clean the potatoes and pour them into the still cold water, bring to a boil, and cook for about 5/7 minutes, no longer because they must remain crispy. Cool and cut into slices.
Cut the onion after peeling it and cut it into thin strips. Cut the onion after peeling it and cut it into thin strips.. Add the onions and the garlic. Top the vegetables with potato slices. Season boiled potatoes with salt and pepper and cook without stirring for 5-10 minutes. When the onions have begun to caramelize on the bottom of the pan, gently turn the mixture so that the potatoes are on the bottom and the onions are roughly on top.
Cook the potatoes for another 5 or 10 minutes or until they begin to brown, you can add more oil if you feel it is necessary. Continue cooking the potatoes, stirring more frequently until fully cooked.

Nutrition values:
Calories 288,Total Fat 13g,Saturated Fat 1.5g,Sodium 276mg,Total Carbs 41g, Dietary Fiber 4g, Total Sugars 1g

PANCAKES

*By now they have become famous and indispensable in our tables, especially for our breakfast.
When you buy a flour mix, check the ingredients carefully so that they do not contain eggs or dairy products.*

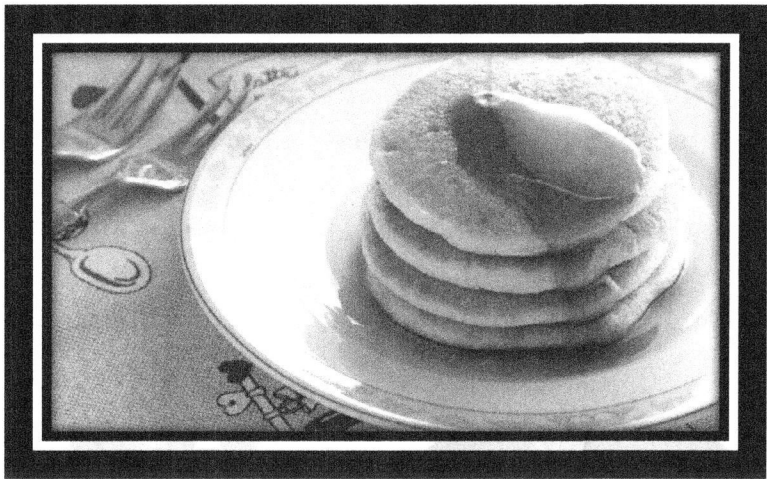

Ingredients:
Servings:4

- 2 cups flour
- ½ cup of apple juice
- 2 tablespoons of canola oil
- Non-stick cooking spray or other oil
- 2 teaspoons baking powder
- ½ teaspoon baking soda
- ¼ teaspoon salt
- 2 tablespoons apple juice or mashed banana
- 1 tablespoon maple syrup

- 1 cup soy milk

Description:

In a medium or large-sized bowl, pour in the flour and mix with baking powder, baking soda, and salt. Add the applesauce, maple syrup, soy milk, apple juice, and canola oil and mix until everything is combined. Take a non-stick skillet or smooth griddle and heat over medium-high heat brush lightly with oil or cooking spray. When the skillet is hot, drop batter by spoonfuls. Bake pancakes until bubbles form on top and edges become firm and golden brown. Flip pancakes over with a rubber spatula and cook on the other side until puffy and golden brown on the bottom.
Serve immediately to savor the fragrant flavor.

Nutrition values:
Calories:128,Fat 3.57g, Carbs 19.41g, Protein 4.33g

CREPES

The trick to making good crepes is to prepare the batter the night before you cook them. This gives the gluten time to develop and prevents the crepes from breaking.
The tools for making great crepes are a non-stick pan and a heat-resistant rubber spatula.

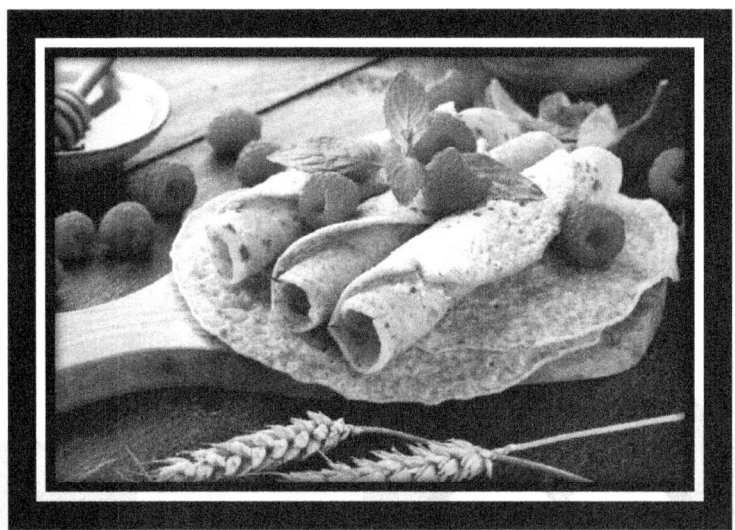

Ingredients:
Servings: 4

- Non-stick cooking oil or spray
- One tablespoon potato starch
- 1 cup flour
- ½ teaspoon salt
- 2 tablespoons vegan margarine, melted
- ½ cup soy milk

Description:

Combine the dry ingredients in a bowl, and with a wooden spoon, stir ¾ cup of water into the dry ingredients. The dough will be firm and a little difficult to work with but go ahead because it is essential to the success of the recipe. Combine the margarine into the dough.

Gradually add the soy milk. When the mixture has become a thick batter, mix until the batter is smooth. Cover the batter and let rest at least 2 hours at room temperature or for 6 hours or more in the refrigerator. To cook the crepes, heat the pan over medium heat for a few minutes.

When the skillet is very hot, turn the heat to high. Lightly brush the bottom of the skillet with oil or cooking spray. Hold the skillet at a 45° angle to the stove. Place a ladleful of batter in the bottom of the skillet.

To distribute the batter evenly, quickly tilt the pan in a circular motion.. The batter will cook as it hits the pan. When an even layer of batter covers the bottom of the pan, return the pan to heat.

Cook crêpe for about 2/3 minutes or until small bubbles form on top.

Turn the crepe with a rubber spatula and cook the other side for about a minute or until lightly browned. Once cooked, place crepes on a tray and cover with a cloth to keep warm

Nutrition values:
Calories: 50, Saturated Fat: 0.4 g, Dietary Fiber: 0.2 g
Total Fat: 1.3 g

WAFFLES

WAFFLE is a waffle cake, originally from Northern Europe, crispy on the outside and soft on the inside, baked-on double hot plates that give it the characteristic lattice-like appearance

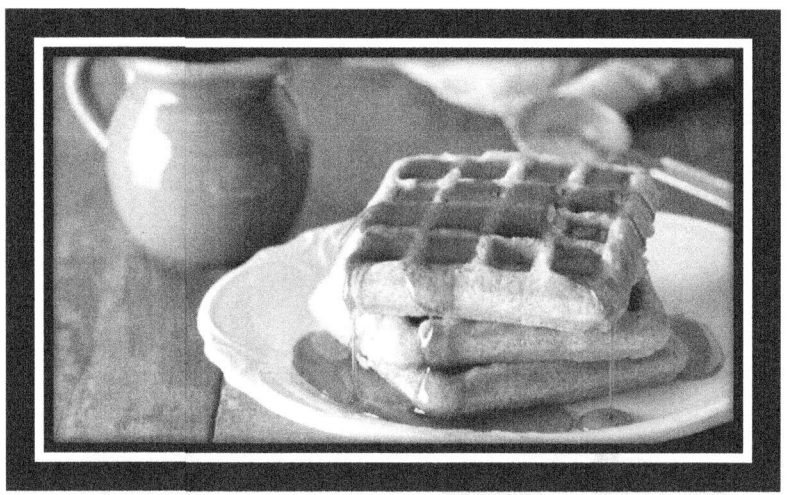

Ingredients:
Servings:2

- Two teaspoons sugar
- ½ teaspoon salt
- 1 tablespoon egg replacer mixed with ¼ cup water
- 1 cup soy milk
- 2 tablespoons oil
- 1 cup whole wheat pastry flour
- ½ cup all-purpose flour
- 1 tablespoon baking powder
- Non-stick cooking spray or other oil

Description:

In a relatively large bowl, whisk together the egg replacer, soy milk, and oil. Stir in the dry ingredients until smooth and homogeneous. Then spray waffle iron with cooking spray or brush with oil and heat over medium heat. Pour in batter until it fills the griddle. Close and cook until the waffle has puffed up and steam no longer escapes from the sides.
You will get eight waffles.

Nutrition values:
Calories: 278.9, Sodium: 885.2 mg, Dietary Fiber: 8.8 g Monounsaturated Fat: 3.5 g

GOOD MORNING MUFFINS

This muffin recipe will give you a nice boost of energy and a good mood to start your day off right.

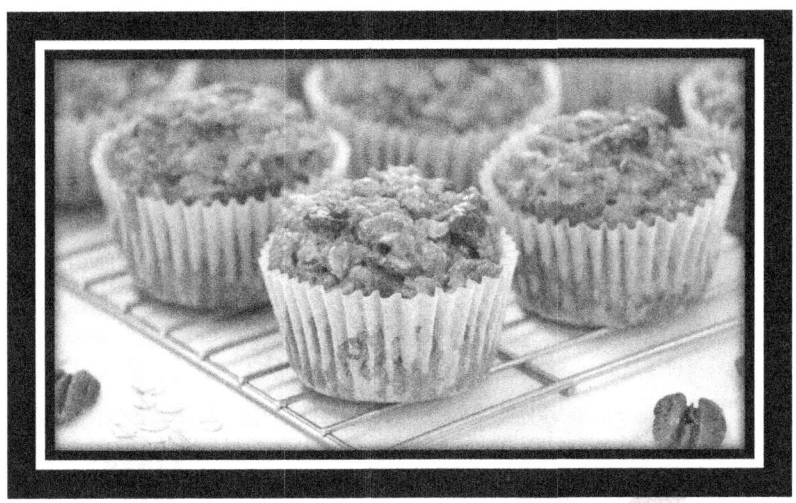

Ingredients:
Servings:2

- 1 cup all-purpose flour
- 1 tablespoon baking powder
- ½ teaspoon cinnamon powder
- ½ teaspoon salt
- ½ cup sugar
- ½ cup raisins
- ¼ teaspoon nutmeg powder
- ¼ teaspoon mace powder
- 2 tablespoons flaxseed
- ¼ cup molasses
- ½ cup apple juice
- 1 cup soy milk

- ¼ cup oil
- 1 cup whole wheat pastry flour
- ¼ cup soy flour

Description:

Preheat oven to 380°. Spray a nonstick baking sheet (for 12-cup muffins) with cooking spray; insert paper liners into cups.
In a medium bowl, combine the different flours, baking powder, cinnamon, nutmeg, mace, salt, and sugar.
Pour in the raisins and stir to coat the flour mixture. Whisk flax seeds with two tablespoons of water. In a small bowl, whisk the molasses, pureed flaxseed, and applesauce until well combined. Whisk in the Soy milk and oil into the applesauce mixture.
Add the wet ingredients to the dry ingredients and mix just until the mixture is blended. Fill muffin pans two-thirds full. Bake for 20-25 minutes.

Nutrition values:
*Calories: 198kcal Carbohydrates: 28g Protein: 3g :
Sodium: 220mg Potassium: 135mg
Fiber: 3g Sugar: 12g*

CONCLUSIONS

The vegan breakfast is a healthy breakfast that helps to preserve the body from many diseases and at the meantime gives our body a valid sustenance in terms of both calories and energy. Very useful to face the day until the next meal, mid-morning snack or lunch.

So from the point of view of taste, the vegan breakfast diet is not affected compared to the traditional breakfast. In fact, I would say that there are much tastier vegan foods as well as excellent to give our body the daily ration of what we need to start great another day.

APPETIZER AND SNACKS

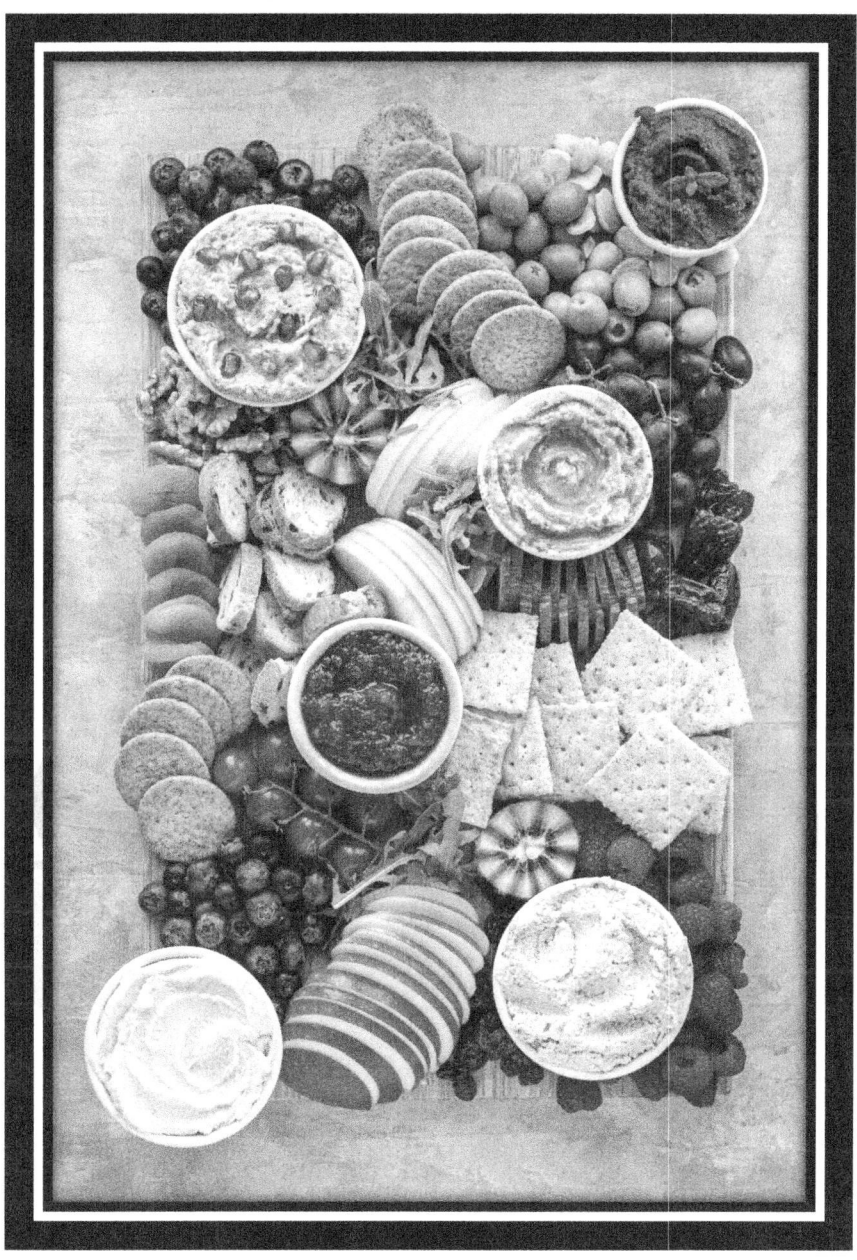

PREVIEW

Good vegan appetizers wanted?

Yes, because it is not apparent that during a vegan dinner is given due attention to this category, generally mistreated.

Vegan appetizers can really be the gem of a dinner or lunch: you can launch into ethnic reinterpretations, try your hand at "alternative" meatballs or delicious salads, or take the opportunity to prepare some delicacies a little more caloric than usual.

Get into it with these recipes for vegan appetizers and snacks, and remember that, especially with vegan cooking, there are really no limits to imagination.

I have selected several recipes for you, so have fun and again choose a recipe to your liking per day for 28 days. I'm sure you will be surprised by the taste and the results you will get.

TUSCAN WHITE BEAN SPREAD

We use very fruity olive oil in this recipe. If you want a more robust flavor, you can add some raw garlic. You can also add some of your favorite hot sauce.
Spread it on some good Italian bread and garnish with roasted red peppers, fresh tomato slices, or grilled portobello for an easy but elegant appetizer.
Use fresh sage leaves as a garnish.

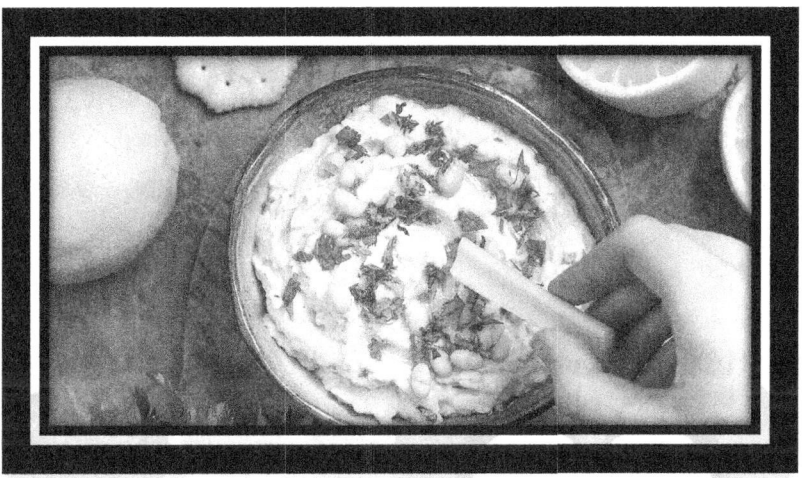

Ingredients:
Servings:4/6

- 2 cups cooked white beans
- 1 teaspoon oil
- 2 tablespoons extra virgin olive oil
- 1 tablespoon chopped fresh sage
- 2 small onions, thinly sliced
- 4 garlic cloves, thinly sliced
- 1 tablespoon lemon juice

- Sea Salt

Description:

Blend the beans (Cannellini)in a food processor. Take a non-stick skillet and heat the oil.
Add the onions and garlic, and constantly stir until the onions turn golden brown.
To the beans pureed in the food processor, add the cooked onions and garlic, lemon juice, and olive oil.
Take a kitchen robot or a mixer, combine and mix all the ingredients, then add the sage and sea salt to taste. If necessary, taste and adjust salt and seasoning, add water if it seems too thick and your liking.
You'll get about two cups of sauce.

Nutrition values:
Calories: 34.5 Protein: 2.4 g Dietary Fiber: 1.9 g Vitamin E: 0.1 %

BLACK BEAN DIP

Chipotles are dry, smoky jalapeños that add a warm, smoky dimension and complement the deep, earthy flavors of black beans. If you prefer a milder flavor, the recipe works just as well without them.

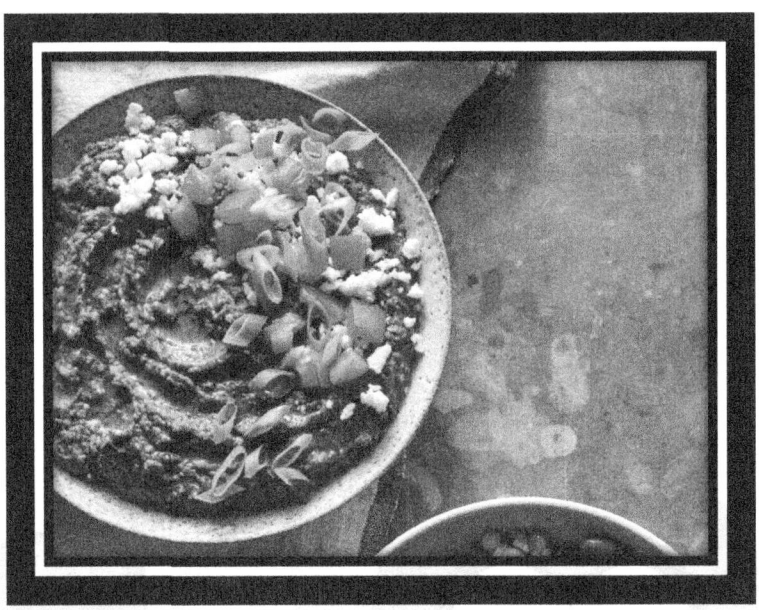

Ingredients:
Servings:4/6

- 4 cups cooked black beans
- One teaspoon oil
- ¼ teaspoon cumin seeds
- 1 small onion, diced
- 1 clove of garlic, minced
- 1/2 teaspoon chili powder
- 1 chipotle chili, canned or dried,
- 2 tablespoons lime juice

- 2 tablespoons fresh chopped cilantro
- Sea Salt

Description:

Puree black beans with a food processor. Heat in a saucepan over high heat in a nonstick skillet. Add the cumin seeds, onion and minced garlic and cook until the onion begins to soften. Add the chili powder and stir well. Cook just until the onion is soft. Add the mixture along with the chipotle beans, lime juice, and cilantro. For a smoother sauce, blend the mixture. Add sea salt to taste and adjust seasonings. Adjust density with water.

Nutrition values:

Calories 704 kJ / 169 kcal, Protein 12 g, Carbohydrates 11 g, Fat 15 g, Fiber 6 g

CURRIED LENTILS DIP

You can add some tomato puree, in which case the whole thing is good on sandwiches with fresh onion and tomato.

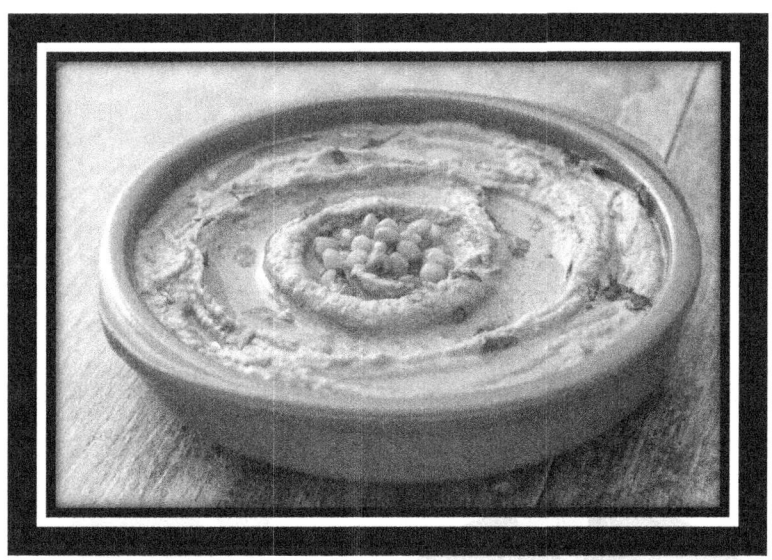

Ingredients:
Servings:4

- Two teaspoons oil
- teaspoon dry mustard or ¼ teaspoon crushed red pepper
- teaspoon white pepper
- 2 cups cooked yellow or red lentils
- 2 tablespoons lemon juice
- 2 tablespoons tahini
- Sea salt
- 1 small onion, diced
- 4 cloves garlic, minced

- 2 teaspoons fresh grated ginger
- 1 teaspoon curry powder
- ½ teaspoon ground cumin
- ¼ teaspoon ground coriander
- teaspoon white pepper

Description:

In a big or large non-stick frying pan, heat oil over medium-high heat. Add the onion, garlic, and ginger. Add the spices and cook for about 4 minutes until the spices start to release their fragrance.
Remove from heat and add the freshly warmed lentils to the pan and mix well.
Mash the lentils with a potato masher or run them through a food processor until coarsely mashed. Add the lemon juice and tahini.
Taste and season with sea salt.
3 cups of sauce.

Nutrition values:
Calories. 80 kCal · Total Carbs. 13 g. Net Carbs. 8 g. Fiber. 5 g. Starch. -. Sugar. 1 g. · Protein. 6 g · Fat. 0.5 g.

GUACAMOLE

There are endless variations on guacamole, but I recommend this simple recipe to allow the avocado flavor to stand out. However, you can add some lovely chopped fresh tomatoes for a touch of color. If you want, you can also add some soy mayonnaise to the guacamole.

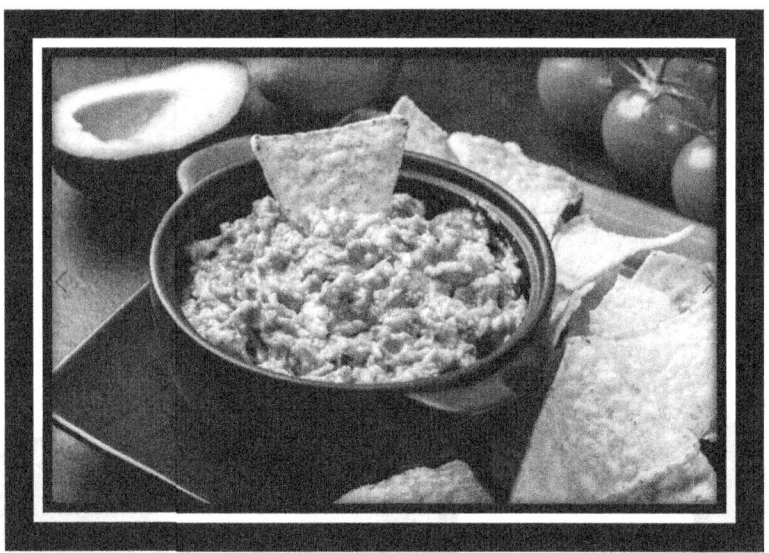

Ingredients:
Servings:6

- 4 ripe avocados
- 1 small jalapeño, fresh or canned, chopped
- 1 tablespoon fresh cilantro, chopped
- Sea salt
- 2 tablespoons lemon juice
- 2 cloves of garlic, minced
- ½ small onion or 4 green onions, thinly sliced

Description:

Mash the avocados with a fork in a small bowl. Add all other ingredients taste, add salt and adjust seasonings to your taste.
With these servings, you will get about 3 cups of guacamole.

Nutrition values:
Calories: 109, Fat: 10g, Sat Fat: 1g, Carbs: 6g, Sodium: 165mg, Fiber: 165mg

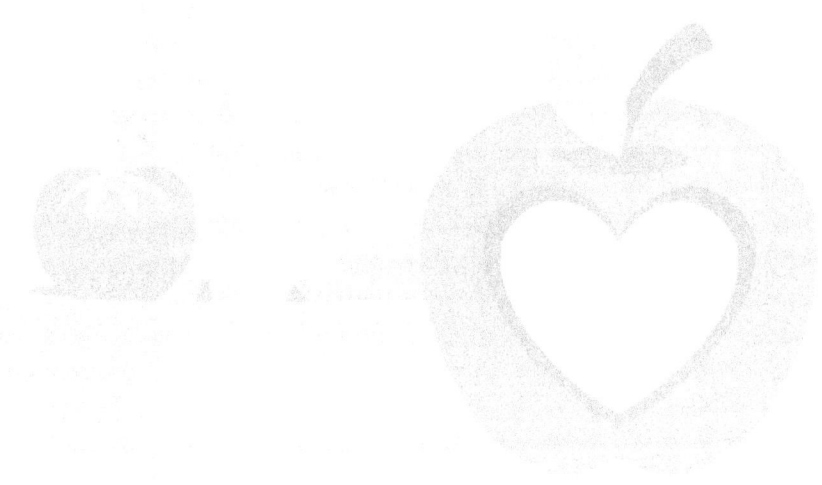

SKORDALIA

Garlic and potatoes are two foods that combined together create a good sauce to serve with raw vegetables or toasted bread triangles.
Also great as a sandwich, with some thinly sliced red onion and grilled vegetables.

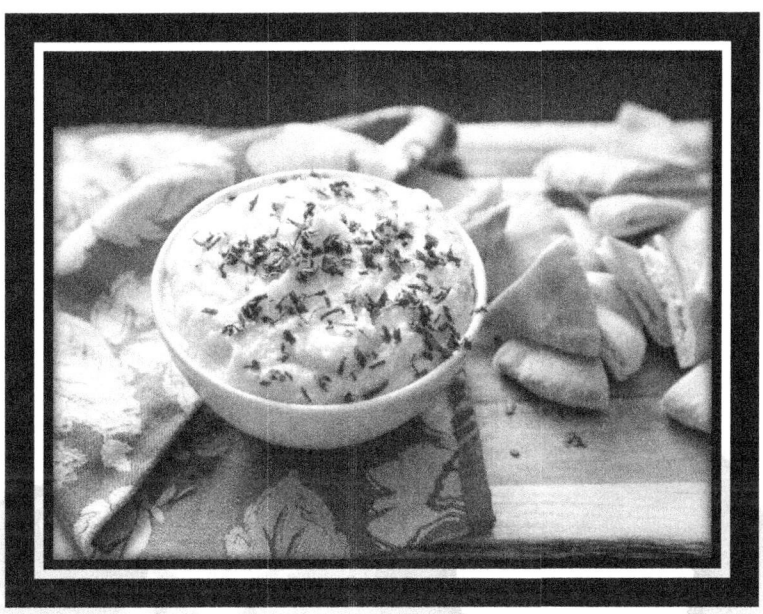

Ingredients:
Servings:4

- 2 cups mashed potatoes
- 1 tablespoon minced garlic
- ½ cup extra virgin olive oil
- 3 tablespoons wine vinegar or lemon juice
- Salt and pepper

Description:

Mix all ingredients in sequence in a medium-sized bowl. Taste the mixture and dose the seasonings with salt and pepper to suit your taste.
The quantity obtained was 3 cups.

Nutrition values:
Calories: 108, Fat: 10g, Sat Fat: 1g, Carbs: 9g, Sodium: 160mg, Fiber: 185mg

CAPONATA

I wish more people loved eggplant! Maybe this recipe It will help make you appreciate these seasonal vegetables. Green olives are usually used; I prefer kalamata. If you can't find good fresh tomatoes, you can use canned diced tomatoes.

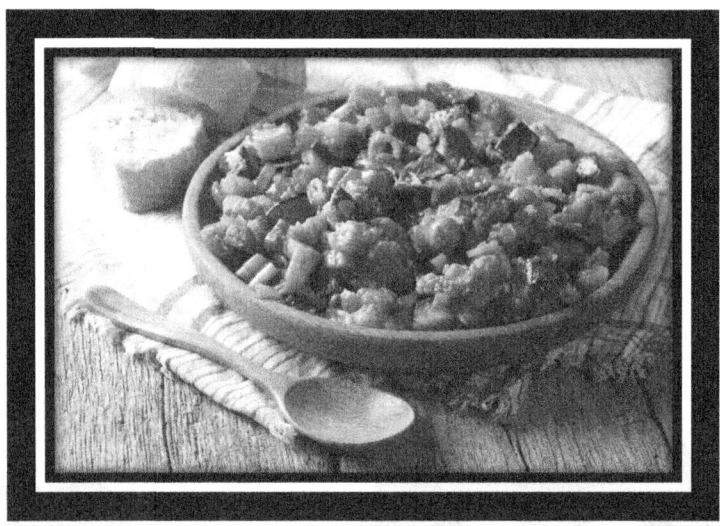

Ingredients:
Servings:4

- Tomatoes.
- 1 pound eggplant, cut into 1-inch cubes
- 6 teaspoons oil
- 3 tablespoons kalamata olives, pitted and chopped
- teaspoon freshly ground black pepper
- 1 celery stalk, cut into rounds
- 1 medium onion, chopped

- 3 garlic cloves, minced
- ½ cup red wine vinegar
- 1 tablespoon sugar
- 1½ cups diced tomatoes with seeds
- 1 tablespoon capers
- 1 tablespoon lightly toasted pine nuts
- 2 tablespoons chopped fresh parsley
- 1 tablespoon fresh basil, coarsely chopped
- Salt

Description:

Generously salt the eggplant cubes and place them in a colander. Allow draining for 30 minutes. Eggplant will release a fair amount of light brown liquid. Rinse briefly under cold water and pat dry.

Heat 3/4 teaspoons oil in a large skillet over medium-high heat. Add the celery, onion, and garlic and sauté until the onion is soft and golden brown. Soop the onions and celery from the skillet and place in a large bowl. Heat another 2 teaspoons of oil in the skillet over medium-high heat. Add the diced eggplant and cook until lightly browned about 10 minutes.

Add the eggplant to the bowl with the onions and celery.

Add the sugar and the vinegar to the pan, bring to a boil and reduce the mixture by half. Pour the vinegar mixture over the eggplant mixture and stir until vegetables are coated. Allow the mixture to cool slightly.

When the all mixture is still warm, add the remaining ingredients. Taste and adjust seasoning with salt. Allow caponata to rest for at least 30 minutes.
Serve cold or at room temperature.

Nutrition values:
Calories: 115.8, Monounsaturated Fat: 2.4 g, Dietary Fiber: 3.7 g, Protein: 2.7 g

TOSTONES

If you are not used to working with bananas, you should know that if they
Are green and a little tricky, they can be fried as tostones (pancakes) or plantain chips, or baked and mashed like potatoes.
This recipe will be a nice twist and will amaze your family and diners.

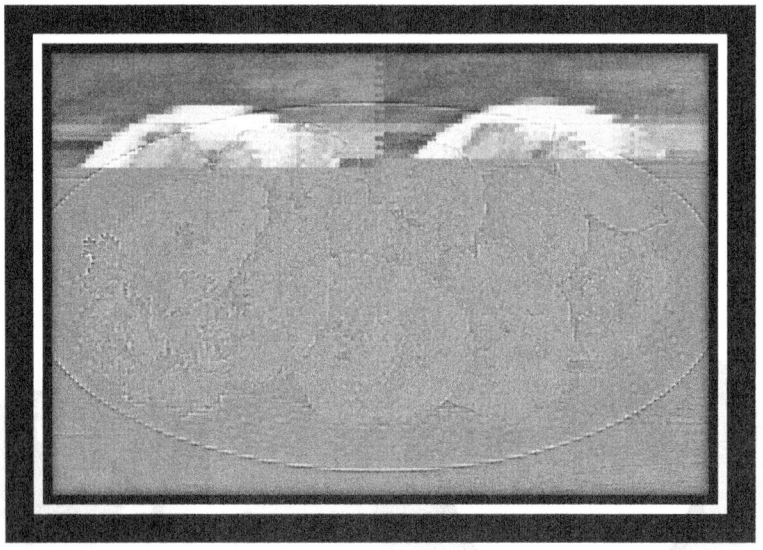

Ingredients:
Servings:6

- 4 plantains, yellow-green and a little hard
- Oil for frying
- Sea Salt
- Pico de Gallo, or canola sauce

Description:

Peel the plantains,and remove the top and bottom with a sharp paring knife. Cut long slits along the plantain, deep enough to go through the peel.
Heat ½ inch of oil in a large skillet over medium-high heat or in a deep fryer at maximum temperature. Cut the bananas into 1-inch slices.
Fry the bananas in a single layer, turning once, for about 2 to 3 minutes
on each side. Remove plantains from oil and drain on a paper towel...
Flatten the slices, which should be about ½ inch thick. If the plantains crumble when flattening, they are not cooked enough so leave them a few minutes longer.
Return the slices to the skillet or fryer and fry until golden brown and crispy.
Season with sea salt. Store in a warm oven or serve immediately with
Accompany with Pico de Gallo or canola sauce.

Nutrition values:
Calories: 11.8, Monounsaturated Fat: 3.4 g, Dietary Fiber: 3.1 g, Protein: 0,5 g

SWEET POTATO FALAFEL

This is a quick recipe that uses a falafel mix, which can be found in most grocery stores. The sweetness of the potato mixes well with the spiciness of the chipotle sauce or Meshwiya.

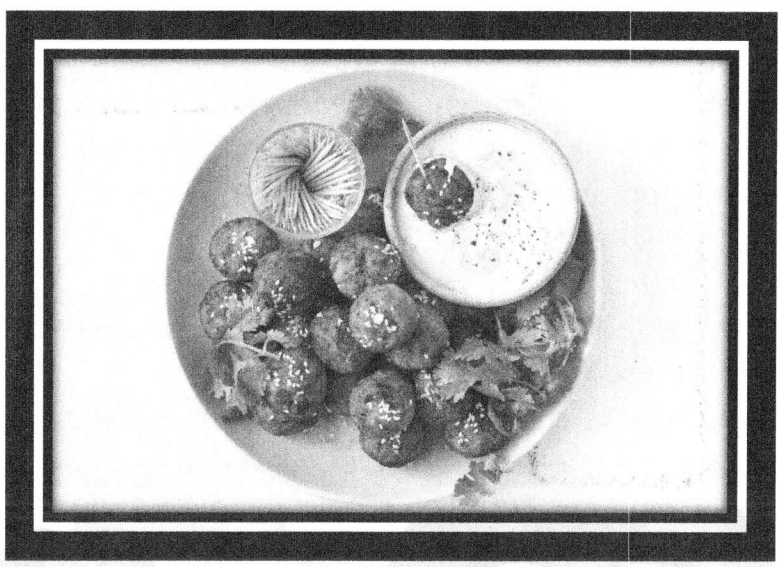

Ingredients:
Servings:4

- 1 cup falafel mixture
- 1 tablespoon chopped fresh cilantro
- 1 teaspoon ancho chili powder
- ½ teaspoon ground cumin
- ¼ teaspoon cayenne
- 1 teaspoon lemon juice
- 1 cup mashed sweet potatoes
- Salt and pepper

- 2 tablespoons oil
- Chipotle or Meshwiya Sauce

Description:

Pour 1 cup boiling water over falafel mixture in a bowl. Cover and let stand for 20 minutes or until the water is absorbed and the ground chickpeas in the mix are soft. Add the cilantro, chili powder, cumin, cayenne, and lemon juice to the falafel mix and mix well. Add the sweet potatoes. Taste the resulting mixture and adjust the seasonings with salt and pepper.
Heat 1 tablespoon oil in a nonstick skillet over medium-high heat. Drop the falafel mix by generous spoonfuls into the pan.
Flatten the falafels with a metal spatula to ensure even cooking and cook for about 3 minutes.
After 3/4 minutes turn the meatballs over and cook the other side for another 3 minutes. Repeat with remaining oil and falafel mixture—season with salt and pepper. Serve immediately.
Serve with Chipotle Salsa or Meshwiya.

Nutrition values:
Calories: 156, Monounsaturated Fat: 2.9 g, Dietary Fiber: 3.2 g, Protein: 2.8 g

VEGAN CHILI RELLENOS

This is a low-fat version. For a more traditional version, you can stuff the peppers with vegan cheese, then flour them with soy milk, flour, and fry them in oil.

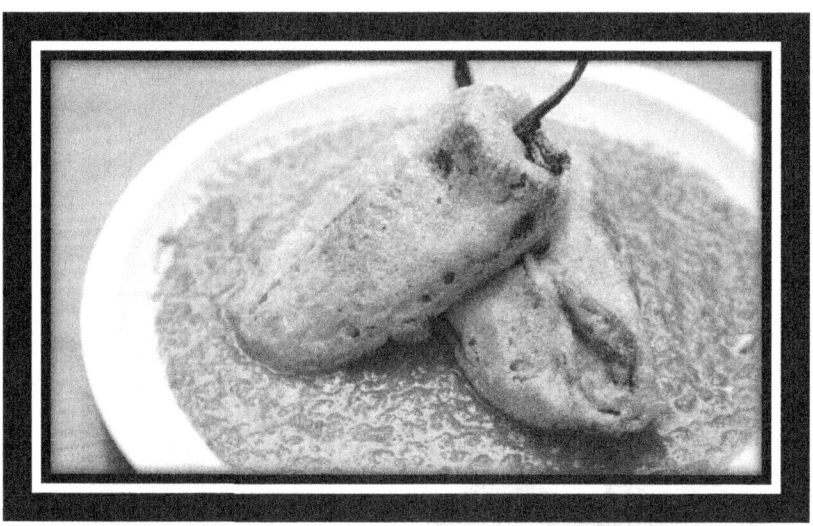

Ingredients:
Servings:4

- 18 jalapeño peppers
- 1 cup slivered almonds
- 1 teaspoon minced garlic
- 1 tablespoon nutritional yeast
- ¾ cup mashed potatoes
- Salt and pepper
- Oil
- Sweet Tomato Sauce

Description:

Preheat oven to 360 degrees. Create with a sharp knife a slit along the side of each bell pepper. Cook the peppers in a pot of boiling salted water for 3-6 minutes. Drain and cool under running water.
Mince the almonds in a spice mill, or chop them very fine with a sharp knife taking care.
Mix the garlic, baking powder, and potatoes with the almonds—season with salt and pepper.
Fill each bell pepper with the mixture. Place the peppers in a well-oiled glass baking dish.
Lightly brush the top of the peppers with oil. Bake the peppers for about 25 minutes. Serve with sweet tomato sauce.

Nutrition values:
392 calories: 63g total carbs, 53g net carbs, 11g fat, 17g protein

CONCLUSIONS

With vegan appetizers, it is possible to find many ideas to start a meal in the best way, in a fresh and healthy way, and without meat or food coming from the animal world, in full respect of vegan and vegetarian standards.

Using ingredients such as tofu, seitan and soy, together with the best of fresh fruit in season and a pinch of creativity, it is possible to prepare easy and tasty appetizers in perfect vegan style, which at the same time are also tasty and appetizing, to satisfy even the most demanding and refined palates.

Among the preparations, there are various appetizers and snacks, snacks for original appetizers.

With the recipes of vegan appetizers and snacks contained in this section, she is accompanied, as always, by photos and simple descriptions, even those who are not experts or beginners in the kitchen can prepare at home with little difficulty delicious and healthy dishes, one hundred percent vegan and natural.

Choose a recipe per day at your leisure and run it for 28 days.

Have fun, explore and eat healthy.

SOUP PASTA AND BREADS

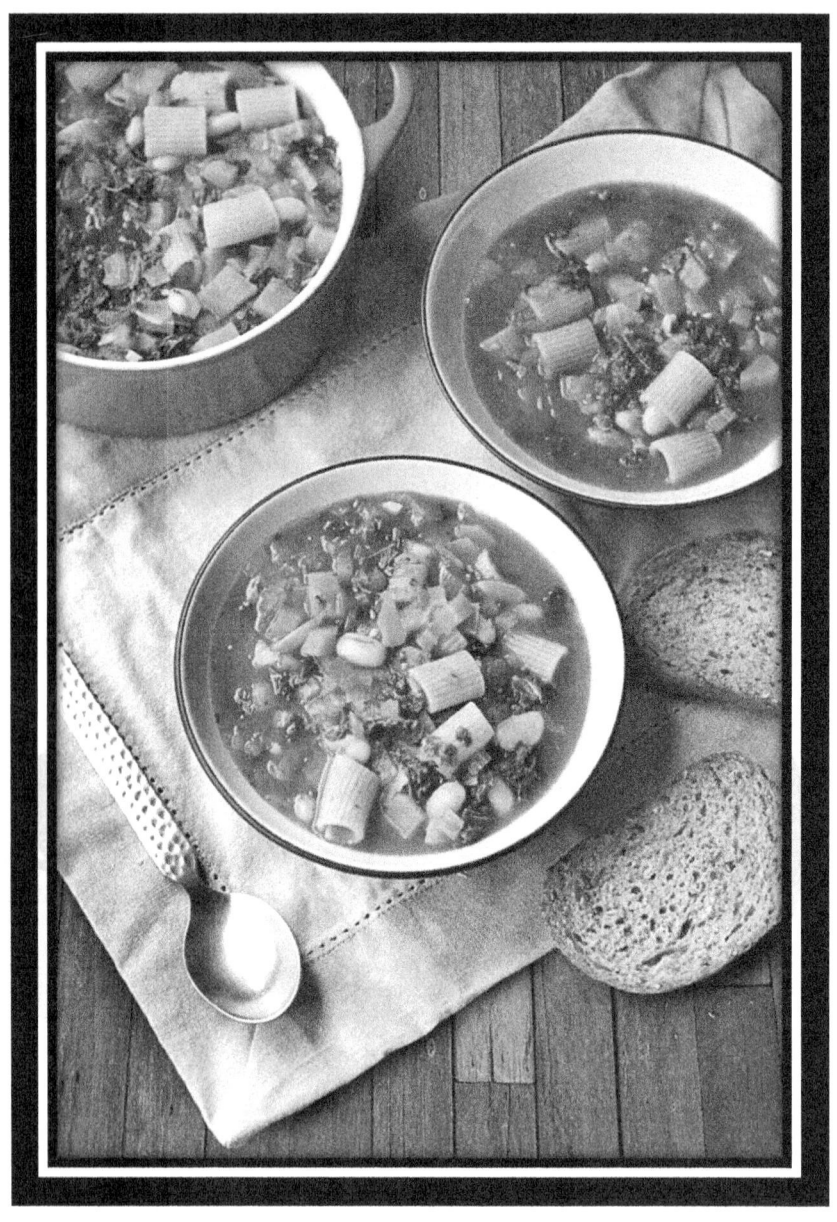

PREVIEW

Do you think that choosing a vegan diet irretrievably means giving up the taste and deliciousness of your dishes? Nothing could be more wrong.

Particularly with regard to the first courses, many typical preparations of the Mediterranean tradition such as pasta, gnocchi, soups, and velvety soups are perfect to be declined in a vegan version without losing anything.

Seasonal ingredients and imagination are the basis for creating a little 100% veg masterpiece every time.

Try the recipes I have prepared below; I'm sure if you have any doubts, you will change your mind.

Let's get started.

VEGETABLE STOCK

Vegetable broth, is so simple and versatile and you'll be amazed yourself.

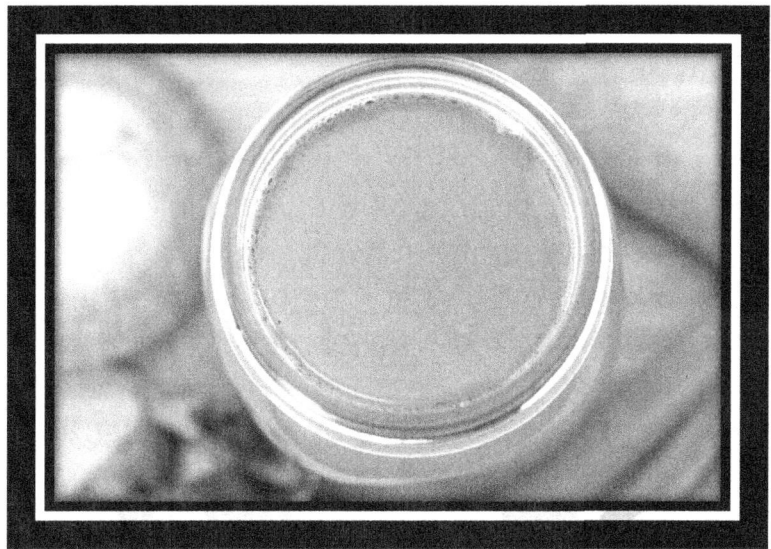

Ingredients:
Servings: 6

- 4 onions, peeled and cut into quarters
- 8 cloves, whole
- 4 celery stalks, cut into 2-inch pieces,
- 4 carrots, cut in half lengthwise, then into 2-inch pieces
- 2 to 4 cups vegetable scraps
- 2 bay leaves
- 4 sprigs of fresh thyme
- 10 garlic cloves, crushed
- 4 black peppercorns

Description:

Take a large pot with 4 liters of cold water and pour all the ingredients and put on the fire at high temperature.
For a stronger, more enveloping flavor, stick a clove into each onion.
When the water is about to boil, lower the heat to medium. Partially cover the pot and simmer the broth for about an hour or until all the vegetables are soft enough. Taste the broth.
To make a light broth, strain the broth through a strainer and mash on the vegetables to extract all the liquid.
If you prefer to have a thicker broth before straining, puree it with an immersion blender. Using a strainer, strain the broth to discard stringy, inedible fibers.
If you want a stronger, more intense flavor and a thicker broth, return the broth to the pot and reduce it to half.

Nutrition values:
11 calories ; Fat · 0.2g ; Saturated Fats · 0.1g ; Cholesterol · 0mg ; Carbohydrate · 2.1g

GREEN VEGETABLE BROTH

This broth is ideal for soups with spring vegetables, such as asparagus and peas Use the central, tender leaves of romaine lettuce , asparagus ends, basil stalks, green beans, broccoli stalks, Chinese cabbage clippings, and the like to flavor this delicate broth.

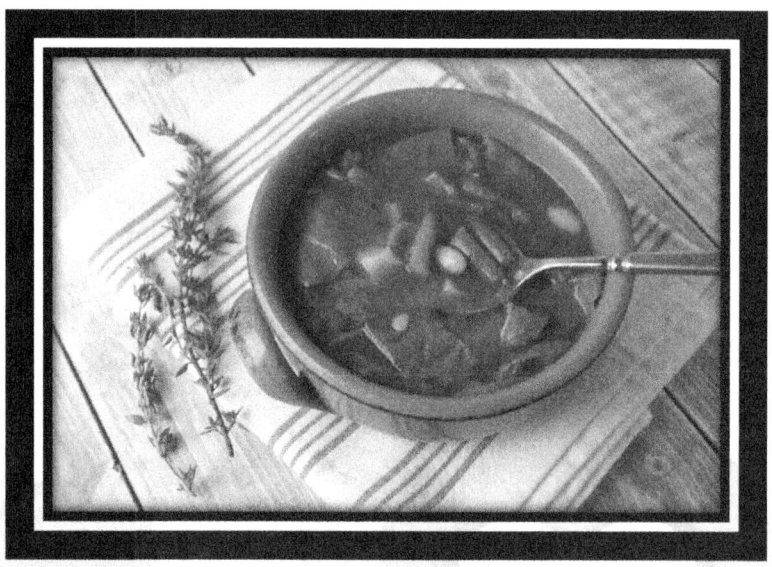

Ingredients:
Servings:4

- 1 bunch of green vegetable scraps
- 1 romaine lettuce, cut into 2-inch squares
- 4 green onions, cut into 4-inch lengths
- 3/4 asparagus
- 1 small bunch of green beans
- 1 stalk of broccoli
- ½ bunch of parsley

- 2 cloves garlic
- 2 bay leaves

Description:

Cover the previously washed vegetables and bay leaves with cold water in an earthenware pot and bring to a boil over high heat.
When water is about to boil, reduce heat to medium. Cook the broth for 20 min.
Remove the crock pot from the heat and let it sit for about 30 minutes.
Strain the broth through a large hole strainer. Press gently on the vegetables to extract all the broth. Discard the solids.

Nutrition values:
18 calories; Fat 0.5g ; Saturated Fats 0.2g ; Cholesterol 0mg ; Carbohydrate 2.6g

MISO SOUP

This is a slightly more complex version, but all miso soups quickly prepare.

Dark miso is saltier than light miso, so adjust the flavor with soy sauce as you prefer. In Japan, this soup is eaten for breakfast, while I like it for dinner.

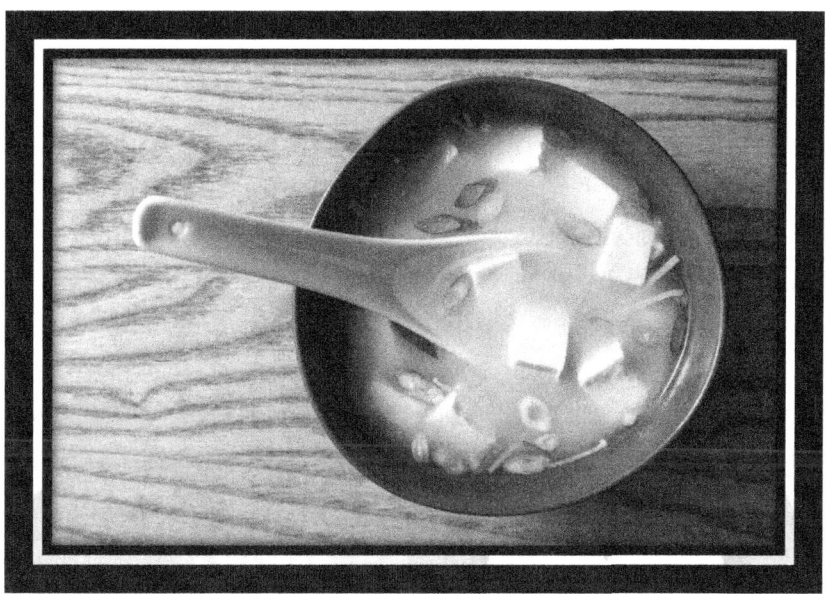

Ingredients:
Servings:6

- 4 cups of Japanese seaweed broth
- 1 teaspoon minced garlic
- ½ medium onion, thinly sliced
- 1½ teaspoons fresh grated ginger
- ½ cup matchstick-cut carrots
- 1 cup thinly sliced button mushrooms
- 1 3-inch piece of wakame

- 2 thinly sliced green onions
- 1 cup thinly sliced seasonal vegetables (asparagus, green beans, watercress, dandelion)
- 5 tablespoons miso
- 10 ounces tofu, cut into small cubes

Description:

Pour the broth into a soup or soup pot, add the garlic, onion, ginger, carrots, mushrooms, and seaweed. Bring to a boil over high heat. Reduce the to medium heat and simmer for about 5 10 minutes until the carrots are tender.

Add the green onions and seasonal vegetables. Simmer for another 8 minutes or until vegetables are crisp and tender. In a small bowl, slowly add 1 cup of broth to the miso and whisk until there are no more lumps. Add the miso and tofu to the soup.

Cover the crockpot with a lid and let it stand by turning off the heat. Pour the resulting soup into individual covered bowls and let steep for 3 to 4 minutes.

Nutrition values:

87 calories.7.2g total carbs, 5.5g net carbs, 3.5g fat, 6g protein

ONION SOUP

This soup can satisfy the most nostalgic palates of French-style onion soup. Feel free to top the soup with a large crouton and some vegan cheese. Delicious I assure you, especially on winter evenings.

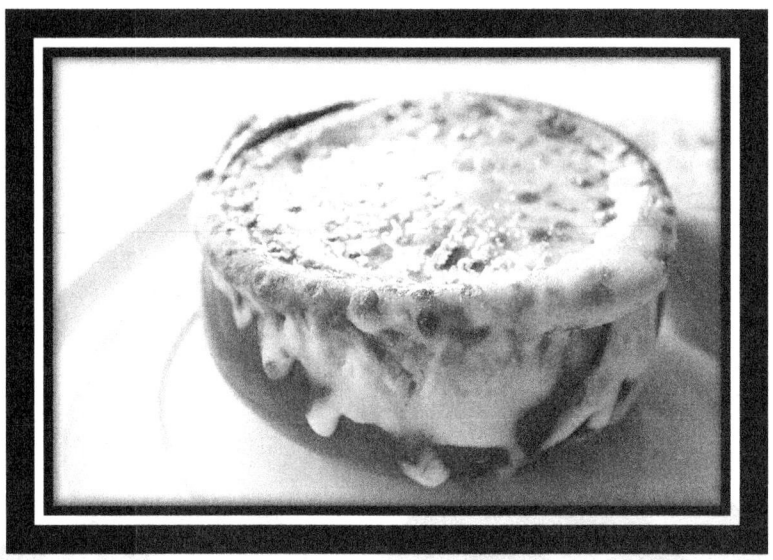

Ingredients:
Servings:6

- 1 tablespoon oil
- 4 onions, cut in half and sliced ½ inch thick
- 3 garlic cloves, chopped
- 2 teaspoons fresh thyme leaves
- 4 cups mushroom broth
- 2 teaspoons of Spike seasoning
- Sea salt and pepper

Description:

In a large soup pot possibly made of earthenware, heat the oil over medium heat. When the oil begins to smoke, add the onions, garlic and fresh thyme. Cook without stirring until the onions develop some color, about 2 minutes, and then stir. Cook, stirring every 2 minutes until the onions are a deep brown color.
Be careful not to let the onions blacken too much. When most of the onions have turned a rich brown color, add the broth, fresh thyme and Spike.
Raise the heat to a boil. Reduce heat to medium.
Taste the soup and adjust seasonings.

Nutrition values:
86 calories.5.2g total carbs, 2.5g net carbs, 1.5g fat, 0,2g protein

.

LENTIL AND SPINACH SOUP

This lentil soup is really delicious and can be made with either vegetable stock or water. If you use water, you will have a more concentrated flavor, and the taste of the lentils will be stronger.

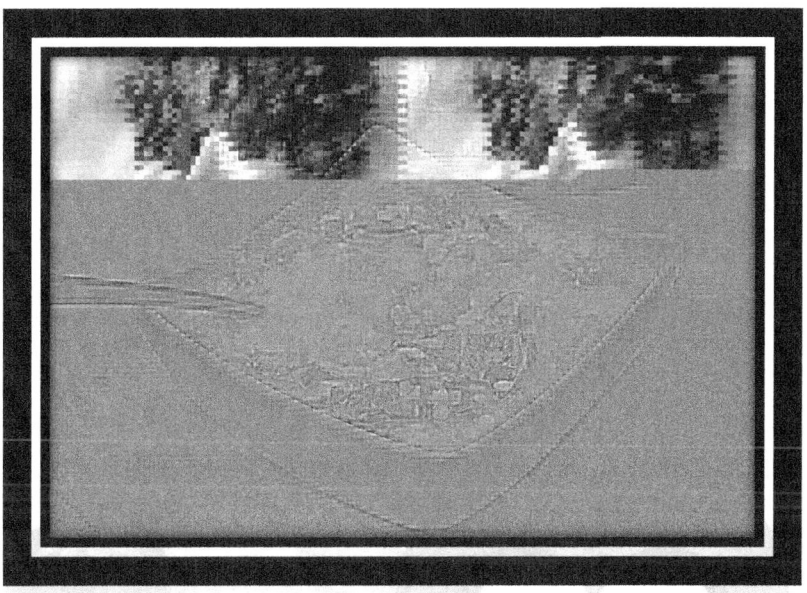

Ingredients:
Servings:2

- 1 tablespoon oil
- 2 cups brown lentils, washed
- 1 teaspoon salt
- ¼ teaspoon black pepper
- 4 cups spinach leaves, washed and coarsely chopped
- 2 medium onions, diced
- 1 teaspoon minced garlic

- 4 celery stalks, plus hearts, diced
- 2 medium carrots, diced
- 1½ teaspoons dried basil
- ½ teaspoon dried thyme
- 1 large bay leaf

Description:

Pour the oil and heat in a soup pot over medium-high heat and sauté the onions, garlic,, celery, carrots, and dried herbs until they begin to soften. Pour the oil and heat in a soup pot over medium-high heat and sauté the onions, garlic,and 2 quarts of water or vegetable broth to the pot. Turn the heat up to high and bring the soup to a boil.
Cook lentils for about 20 minutes on low heat until tender.
Add the salt, pepper, and spinach and mix well.
Remove the bay leaf.
Taste the soup and adjust the seasonings. Serve immediately.

Nutrition values:
192 calories, 113 mg of sodium, 15 gr of fiber, 18 gr of protein

ORECCHIETTE WITH BUTTERNUT SQUASH

*Orecchiette is a type of pasta that holds its surge well, and this recipe with pumpkin will be a great find.
If you have difficulty peeling the squash, place it in the microwave for easy cleaning as it softens the skin.*

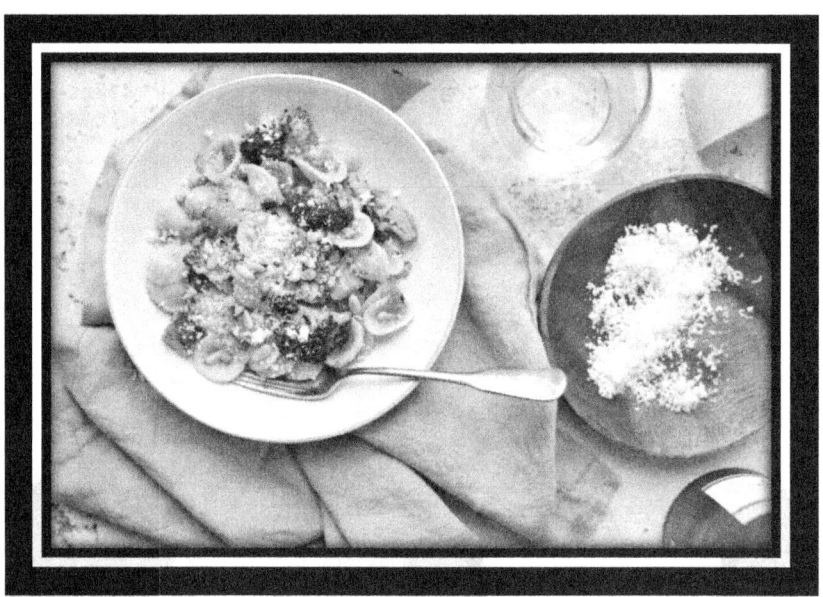

Ingredients:
Servings: 6

- 1 pumpkin, peeled cut into ¾ inch cubes
- 8 ounces of orecchiette pasta
- 4 garlic cloves, thinly sliced
- 1 cup moderately dry white wine
- 2 teaspoons oil
- 1 large leek, white part only, cut in half lengthwise, then sliced

- ½ cup of vegetable stock, or 1 cup of the pumpkin cooking water
- Salt and pepper
- 2 tablespoons extra-virgin olive oil
- 1 tablespoon fresh thyme or dried thyme

Description:

Pour the pumpkin cubes into a pot with about 3 quarts of salted boiling water and cook for a few minutes (max 5 min) until the pumpkin is tender. Drain the squash in a colander and set aside 1 cup of the cooking water (it will be useful in the sauce) and rinse lightly with cold water and set aside in a bowl.

Bring few quarts of water to a boil in a large pot and pour in the orecchiette pasta, which you will cook for about 8 minutes, leaving it al dente.

Using a colander, drain pasta, rinse in cold water to cook it, and set it aside.

Sauté leek and garlic with oil in a large skillet over medium-high heat until leek is soft. Add the dried thyme to the pan with the leeks.

Turn up the heat and add the white wine until it evaporates. Add the vegetable broth or squash cooking water.

Cook until the liquid is reduced by one-fourth. Add the squash to the pot.

Reduce the heat to medium. Taste the resulting sauce and adjust the seasoning to your taste with salt and pepper.

Add the olive oil, fresh thyme, and orecchiette pasta and mix well. Serve immediately.

Nutrition values:
223 calories,40.9g total carbs, 46g net carbs, 2.9g fat, 6.2g protein

AVOCADO SOUP

I personally prefer Hass avocados because of their flavor, and the texture of the flesh is creamy and buttery, light yellow in color. Smooth-skinned Florida avocados are less reliable. But you will be able to get a good result with both.

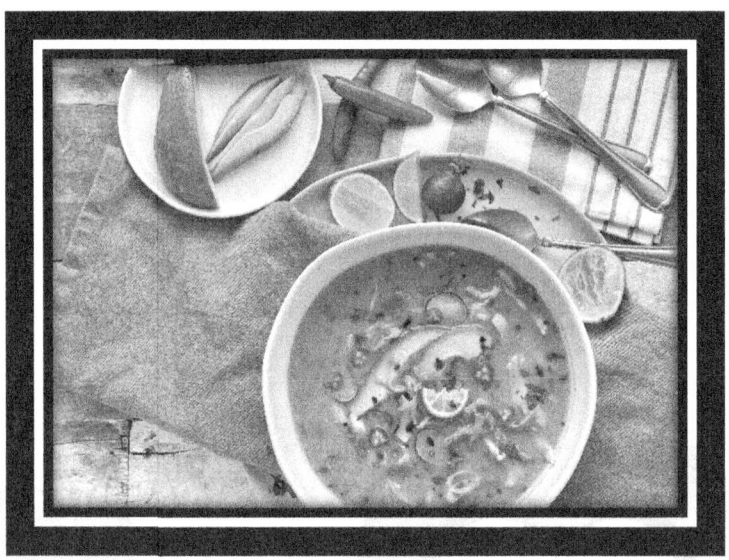

Ingredients:
Servings:6

- 8 ripe Hass avocados or 5 large Florida avocados
- juice of 1 lemon
- 1 teaspoon minced garlic
- 1 small onion, finely chopped
- 1 jalapeño, seeded and chopped
- ¼ cup fresh cilantro, chopped
- 1 tablespoon fresh basil, chopped
- Salt and pepper

- 1 tomato, seeded and diced
- Whole cilantro leaves

Description:

Peel the avocados and scoop out the seeds. In a fairly large bowl, mash the avocados well. Stir in lemon juice, garlic, onion, jalapeño, chopped cilantro and basil. Blend using an immersion blender with cold water until desired consistency is reached, about 3 cups—season with salt and pepper.
Just before serving, toss the tomato with half of the lemon zest. Season with salt and pepper the tomato mix. Add the remaining zest to the soup. Pour the soup into bowls and garnish with the diced tomato mixture or whole cilantro leaves.

Nutrition values:
93 calories, 0.9g total carbs, 16g net carbs, 2g fat, 0.2g protein

FARFALLE WITH SUN DRIED TOMATOES AND PORTOBELLO

This pasta with fresh basil and sun-dried tomato pesto will keep your diners happy...
If you prefer, you could add or replace the mushrooms with broccoli...

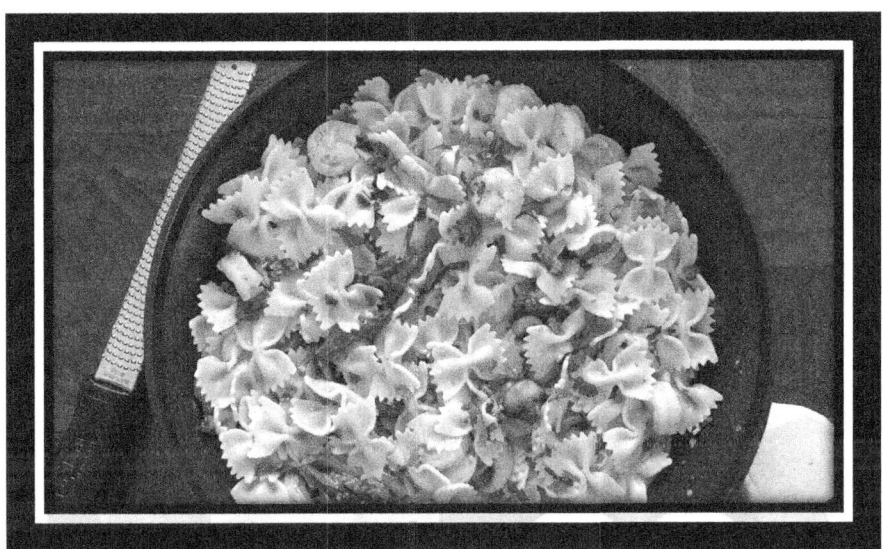

Ingredients:
Servings: 4

- 8 ounces of farfalle (butterfly pasta)
- 2 teaspoons oil
- 1 red onion, cut in half lengthwise
- 3 garlic cloves, thinly sliced
- 3 portobello mushrooms, stemless, thinly sliced
- 1 cup sun-dried tomato pesto
- 1/2 cup basil, thinly sliced

- 1 teaspoon fresh thyme or lemon thyme

Description:

Cook the pasta(farfalle) for about 7 minutes (or according to package directions) in 3 quarts of boiling salted water in a large pot.
Drain with a colander and rinse with cold water to maintain cooking. Pour pasta in a large bowl and let rest.
In a large nonstick skillet, heat the oil over medium heat and add the onion and garlic to and sauté for 3 minutes or just until the onion begins to soften. Add the thinly sliced mushrooms to the skillet and cook for about 4 until soft. Stir gently to avoid breaking the mushrooms. Add the pesto to the skillet along with ½ cup of water. Add the farfalle, mix well and heat through. Add the basil and thyme. Serve immediately.

Nutrition values:
213 calories, 30.9g total carbs, 42g net carbs, 2.5g fat, 6.7g protein

MACARONI AND CHEESE

Macaroni and cheese is a simple dish but at the same time very tasty ...
You can use any type of short pasta.

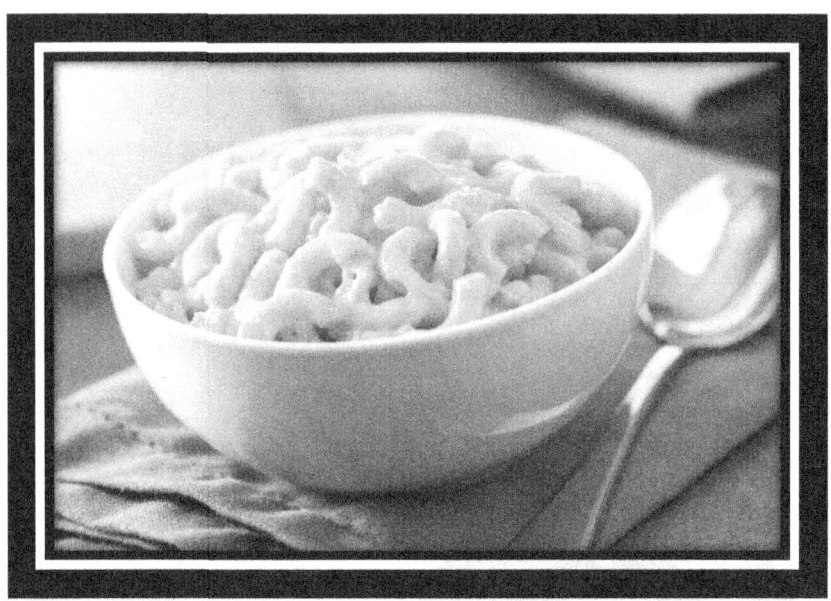

Ingredients:
Servings:4

- 4 cups cooked macaroni
- ¼ cup nutritional yeast
- ½ cup all-purpose flour
- 1 tablespoon light miso
- ½ teaspoon garlic powder
- ¼ teaspoon paprika
- ¼ cup vegan margarine or ¼ cup grape oil
- 2 teaspoons of grainy mustard

Description:

Toast the yeast and flour until the flour begins to brown and the yeast is lightly toasted in a saucepan over medium-high heat. Using a whisk, carefully whisk 2 cups of water (or soy milk) into the flour mixture, be careful not to form lumps
Add garlic powder, miso and paprika, and whisk to mix well. Gently cook the mixture until thick, about 8-10 minutes. Add the margarine and mustard and mix well. Taste and adjust seasonings. Add the previously cooked macaroni and reheat. Serve immediately...

Nutrition values:
300 calories, 6 gr of fat, 48 gr of carbohydrate, 13 gr of protein,

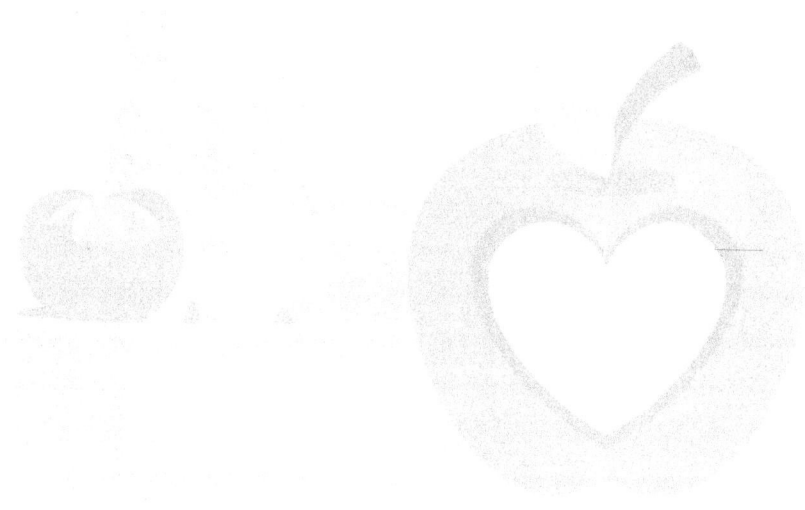

COUSCOUS WITH RAISINS AND PINE NUTS

Couscous can have many variations and goes well with many ingredients, from seasonal vegetables to what you prefer.

Pine nuts can be hard or be very expensive, so substitute slivered almonds.

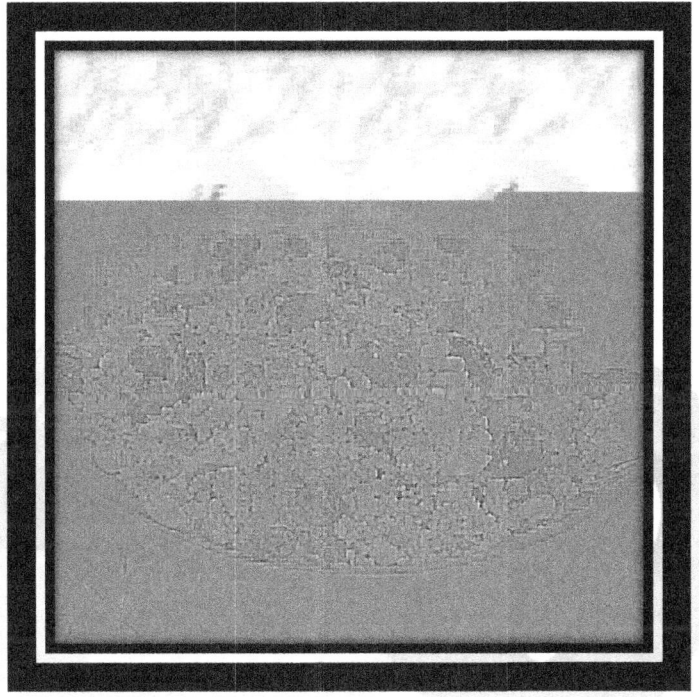

Ingredients:
Servings:4

- 2 cups cooked couscous
- Pinch of nutmeg
- ¼ cup raisins

- 3 tablespoons pine nuts
- 2 teaspoons oil
- 1 medium onion, finely chopped
- ½ teaspoon fresh thyme

Description:

Cover raisins with foil with boiling water in a small cup and let soak for about 10 to 15 minutes.
Over medium heat heat a skillet and pour in the pine nuts and cook, shaking the pan, until the pine nuts are toasted, about 3 minutes. Once golden brown pour the pine nuts onto a plate and set aside.
In the skillet in which you toasted the pine nuts, add the oil and sauté the onion until translucent.
Add the thyme, couscous, and nutmeg and mix well. Remove the raisins from the water with the help of a strainer and add to the couscous. If the mixture is too dry, add three tablespoons of the raisin liquid and stir until absorbed or a drizzle of raw oil.

Nutrition values:
214 calories, 3 gr of fat, 41 gr of carbohydrate, 4,2 gr of protein

POTATO AND ROSEMARY PIZZA

It's very tasty and easy to make, You can use a Taleggio cheese as more flavor and lots of seasoning.

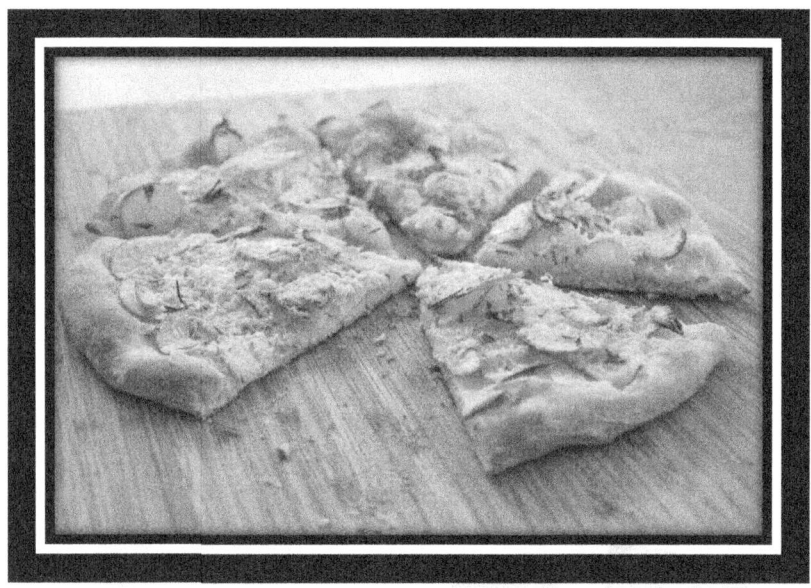

Ingredients:
Servings:4

- 2 pounds new potatoes
- One 12-inch pizza crust, uncooked
- 2 to 3 tablespoons extra virgin olive oil
- 1 teaspoon kosher salt
- 1½ tablespoons chopped fresh rosemary
- Freshly ground black pepper

Description:

Steam the potatoes until they are about halfway cooked. Leave potatoes cool completely. Slice the potatoes thinly on a mandoline or with the side of a grater.
Brush the pizza crust with half of the olive oil. Sprinkle half of the salt and 1 tablespoon of rosemary over the oil. Grind a little black pepper on the crust.
Preheat the oven to 375°. Arrange the potato slices on the pizza up to 1/2 inch from the edge. The potatoes should overlap a bit but should not be more than 2 layers anywhere on the pizza.
Brush the olive oil over the potatoes and sprinkle with the remaining of salt. Bake the pizza in the oven until the potatoes are tender and just begin to brown, about 12 to 15 minutes.
Sprinkle with the remaining rosemary and serve immediately.

Nutrition values:
549 calories, 21 gr of fat, 84 gr of carbohydrate, 1,2 gr of protein

WHITE PIZZA WITH TOFU BOURSIN

For many vegans, white is a favorite pizza that's hard to pass up.

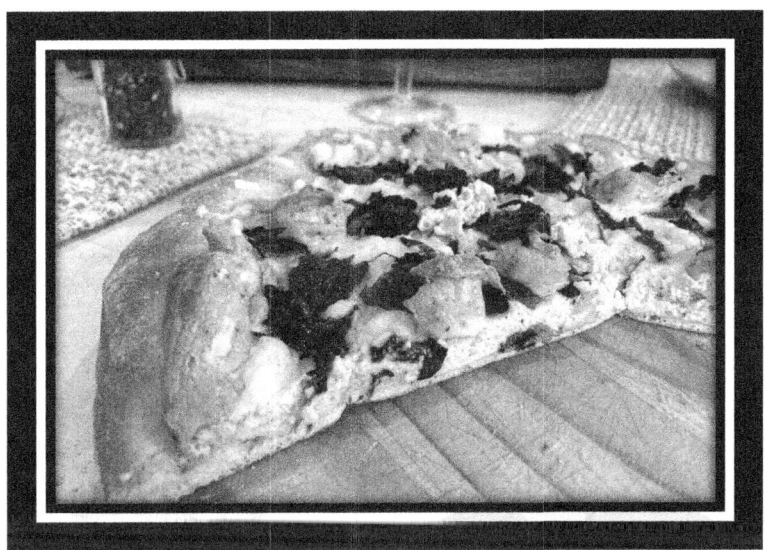

Ingredients:
Servings: 2

- 1 12-inch pizza crust, unbaked
- 1½ tablespoons olive oil
- 2 cups Tofu Boursin
- 1 tablespoon chopped fresh chives
- Freshly ground black pepper
- 2 cups Tofu Boursin
- Freshly ground black pepper

Description:

Preheat oven to 400°. Brush the pizza crust with half of the olive oil. Sprinkle with half of the salt and all of the garlic. Grind some of the black pepper on the crust and spread the Boursin up to ¾ inch from the edge. Using a brush, put the remaining oil on the pizza crust. Bake in the middle part of the oven until the crust begins to brown, about 10-15 minutes. Sprinkle with the remaining salt and chives just before serving.

Nutrition values:
459 calories, 25 gr of fat, 83 gr of carbohydrate, 5,3 gr of protein

RUSTIC PIE

A great idea for reusing leftover grilled vegetables. You can use any type of vegetable any assortment of vegetables, but the ones listed below are a perfect match.

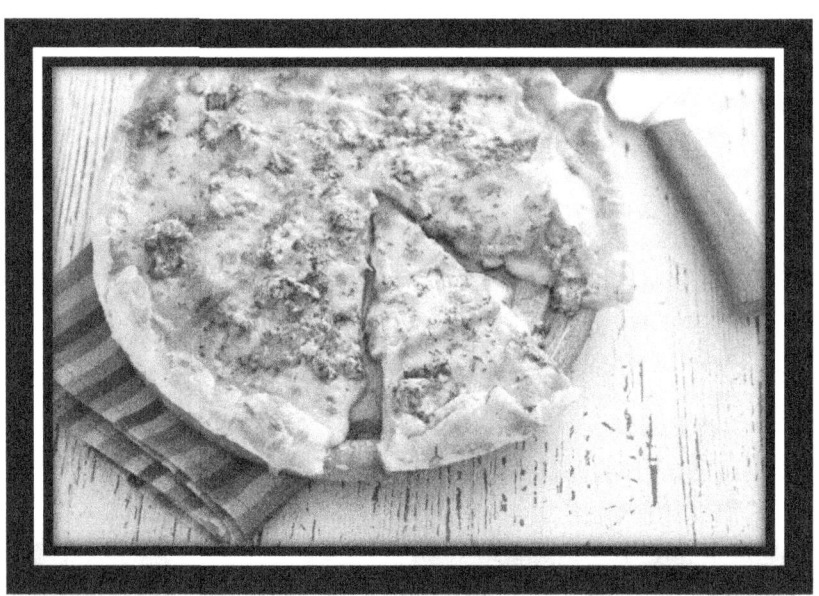

Ingredients:
Servings:4

- 2 12-inch pizza crusts
- 2 tablespoons chopped fresh basil
- 1 teaspoon fresh chopped rosemary
- 1 teaspoon fresh thyme leaves
- 2 tablespoons olive oil
- ¼ teaspoon salt
- 1 teaspoon minced garlic
- Freshly ground black pepper

- 1 medium eggplant, sliced and grilled or roasted
- ¾ cup roasted peppers
- 1 cup Tofu Boursin
- 1 medium zucchini, sliced and grilled or roasted
- 2 medium tomatoes, sliced
- 1 large fennel bulb, thinly sliced and grilled

Description:

Preheat oven to 350°. Roll out one pizza crust 12 inches in diameter and the other other 14 inches. Place the 12-inch crust on a pizza pan.
Mix the basil, rosemary, and thyme in a small bowl. Brush the 12-inch crust with half of the olive oil. Sprinkle the salt, garlic and one-third third of the herbs on the crust. Grind a little black pepper on the crust. Arrange half of the eggplant on the crust, leaving a 2-inch margin around the edge of the pizza. Add half of the roasted peppers and half of the boursin. Layer on all of the zucchini, then the tomatoes. Sprinkle with one-third of the herbs. Cover with all of the fennel, the remaining roasted peppers, the boursin and the eggplant. Sprinkle with the last herbs.
Carefully spread the 14-inch crust over the pie so that the dough comes to inside ½ inch of the bottom edge and gently press down to remove any air pockets. Try to shape the pie so that it is an even height with straight sides. Shape the bottom crust over the top crust together to form an airtight seal all around the

pie. Brush the whole thing with the rest of the olive oil.
Cover the pie with aluminum foil to prevent it from burning too much and bake for 20/25 minutes.

Nutrition values:
470 calories, 21 gr of fat, 56 gr of carbohydrate, 20 gr of protein

CONCLUSIONS

When we find ourselves talking among friends about cooking, whether vegetable or classic, the first question concerns our favorite dish, and usually, the answer is almost never exclusively about cooking.

Much more often, in fact, our preferences include tradition, family, good memories, travel, love, and joy: these are really the ingredients that make up our choice.

So I asked myself, after having forced some of my friends to take part in this little game, what are the ones that most frequently appear on the "lists" of favorite dishes.

Let's start with vegan first courses (of course!); here is my summary.

Now you're spoiled for choice I have prepared several recipes, really all alternative and tasty but above all simple to prepare.

Always be inspired by nature and seasonal produce, as well as yourself, and as always, choose a different recipe from these and run it for 28 days.

VEGETABLE AND SOY FOODS

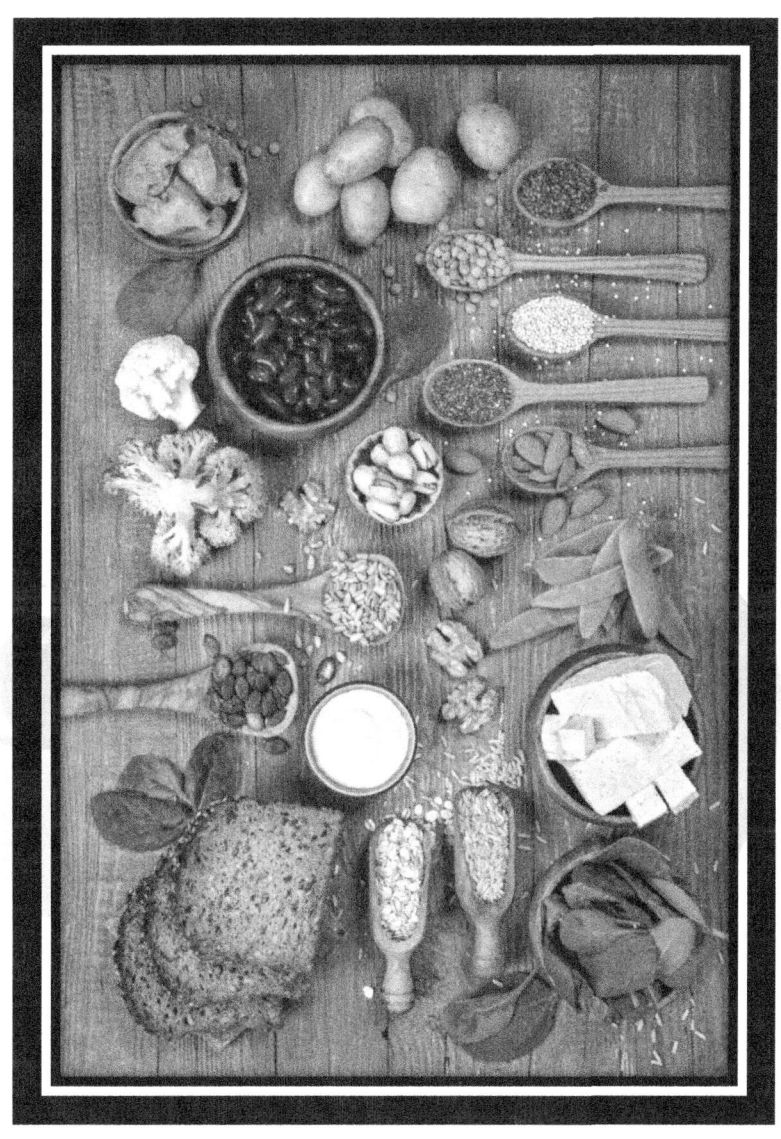

PREVIEW

In recent years, plant-based diets have become very popular, commercial offerings of foods without animal ingredients have also increased.

Soybean is the most common ingredient in plant-based beverages and meat and cheese substitutes due to its high protein content and agricultural production efficiency.

The yellow bean also has a great traditional use among the populations of South-East Asia, where it is consumed in the form of typical foods or as such.

Soy foods are gradually spreading in the West as well, in response to the increasing demand for vegetable foods rich in proteins, especially fed by vegetarians and vegans.

In this section you will find many recipes which I am sure will satisfy your needs.

ARTICHOKE AND ARUGULA SALAD

This salad has a variety of bitter flavors that are well balanced and balanced with the sweetness of bell pepper and mushrooms. Spinach can be substituted for the arugula.

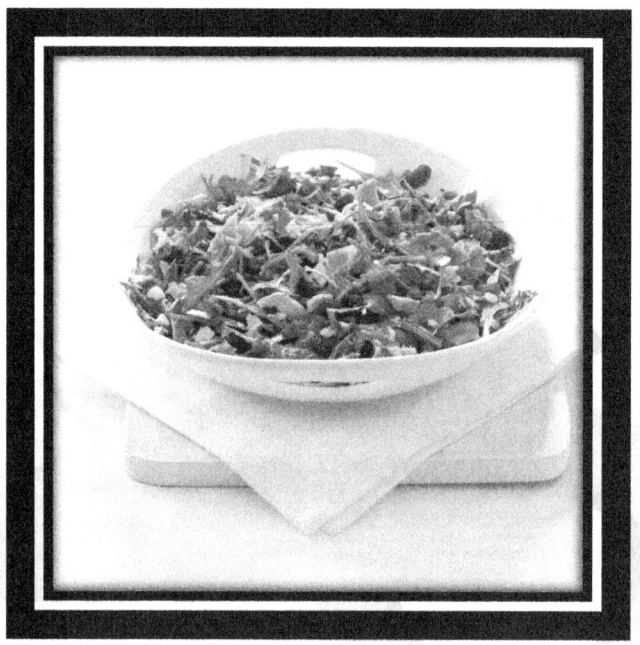

Ingredients:
Servings: 6

- 2 large cleaned artichokes
- 2 tablespoons fresh lemon juice
- ¼ cup extra virgin olive oil
- teaspoon of salt
- Freshly ground black pepper

- 1 red bell pepper, cut into matchsticks
- 1 cup very thin slices of button mushrooms
- 2 tablespoons chopped basil
- 2 bunches of arugula

Description:

In a medium plastic bowl, whisk together the lemon juice, olive oil, salt, and pepper. Pour the artichoke pieces into the dressing immediately after cutting them, so they stay white and don't blacken. Add the bell pepper and mushrooms to the bowl and toss to combine. Let the salad sit for 10 to 15 minutes.
Add the basil and toss a few minutes again before serving.
Divide the arugula among 4 plates salad plates and top with the artichoke salad.

Nutrition values:
169 calories, 13 gr of fat, 12 gr of carbohydrate, 5 gr of protein

GRILLED ASPARAGUS AND LEEKS WITH ALMONDS

This easy roasted asparagus and leek salad recipe makes a perfect spring side dish.

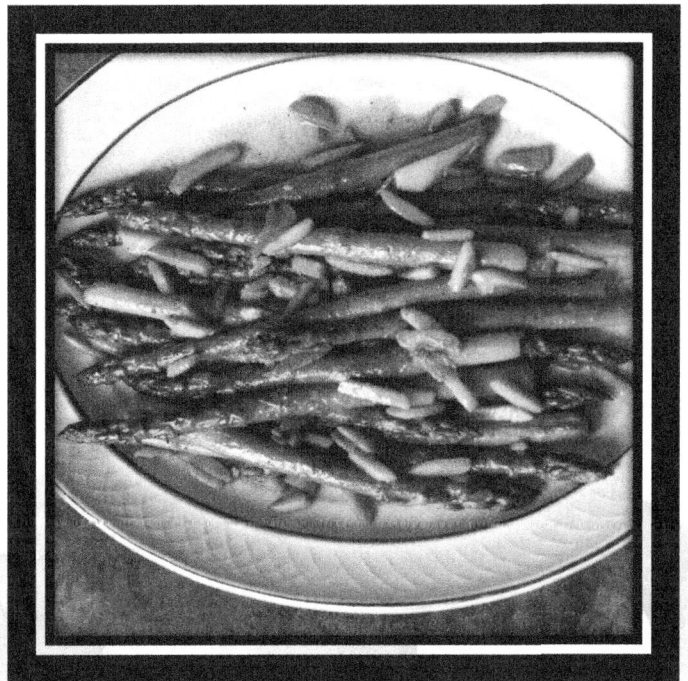

Ingredients:
Servings:4

- 1 large leek
- 1 pound asparagus, blanched
- 1 tablespoon seasoned oil
- Salt and pepper
- ¼ cup mustard-sherry vinaigrette, room temperature

- ¼ cup sliced almonds, toasted

Description:

Simmer leeks for about 5 minutes in salted water until crispy in a large, deep skillet.
Rinse leeks under cold water and pat dry. Cut the leeks in half lengthwise. Rinse well under cold water because there may be sand in them.
Dry thoroughly. Rub the asparagus and leeks with the oil and lightly salt and pepper. Grill the leeks cut side down for a few minutes until heated through. Turn them over and grill the other side. Grill the asparagus until they develop good color. Arrange the vegetables on a platter to a serving dish. Drizzle with the vinaigrette and top with the toasted almonds. Serve immediately.

Nutrition values:
89 calories, 3 gr of fat, 9 gr of carbohydrate, 5 gr of protein,

ROASTED BROCCOLI

This is the best recipe for enjoying broccoli. Roasting intensifies both the sweetness and bitterness of these vegetables and gives them a chewy texture and a slight smokiness. Serve with brown rice and leek tomato sauce.

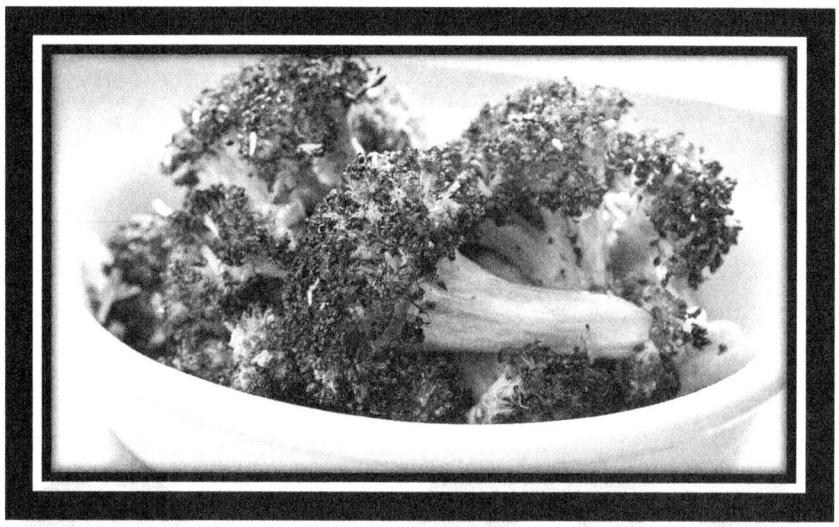

Ingredients:
Servings:4

- 1 head of broccoli, cut into 3-inch florets
- Olive oil
- Salt and pepper

Description:

Preheat oven to 300°. In a small bowl, toss broccoli with enough oil until lightly coated. Season broccoli with salt and pepper.
Take a baking sheet and place the broccoli in a single layer and roast until edges of broccoli begin to brown and stems are tender, about 20 minutes, rotating baking sheet and stirring broccoli halfway through cooking.

Nutrition values:
80 calories, 6 gr of fat, 6 gr of carbohydrate, 3 gr of protein

TUNISIAN CARROT SALAD

Carrots are often not appreciated as much as they should be but I'm sure this recipe will surprise you....

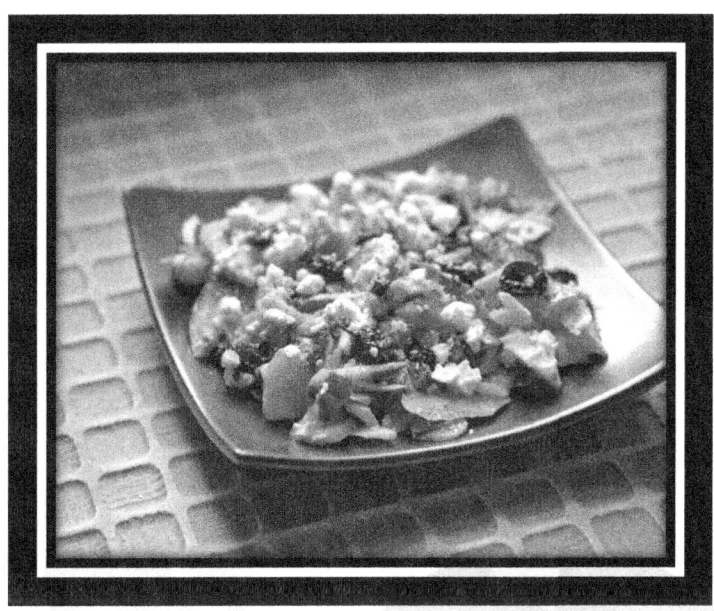

Ingredients:
Servings:4/6

- 2 garlic cloves, crushed
- teaspoon of cayenne
- ½ teaspoon cumin seeds, toasted
- ½ teaspoon ground coriander
- 2 tablespoons lemon juice
- 3 tablespoons extra virgin olive oil
- 4 carrots, shredded or cut into matchsticks
- 2 tablespoons chopped fresh coriander
- Salt and pepper
- 1 head of lettuce, washed and cut

- 4 yellow pear tomatoes, cut in half
- 4 cherry tomatoes, cut in half

Description:

Mix the garlic, spices, lemon juice and olive oil in a medium bowl. Add the carrots and the cilantro and mix well and let stand for 15 minutes.
Taste the salad and season with salt and pepper. Arrange the lettuce on 4 salad plates. Top the lettuce with the carrots. Arrange the tomatoes on the salads. You will get 4 servings.

Nutrition values:
120 calories, 11 gr of fat, 6 gr of carbohydrate, 1 gr of protein

CAULIFLOWER WITH CAPERS

I roasted the cauliflower. This side dish went very well and my guests enjoyed.

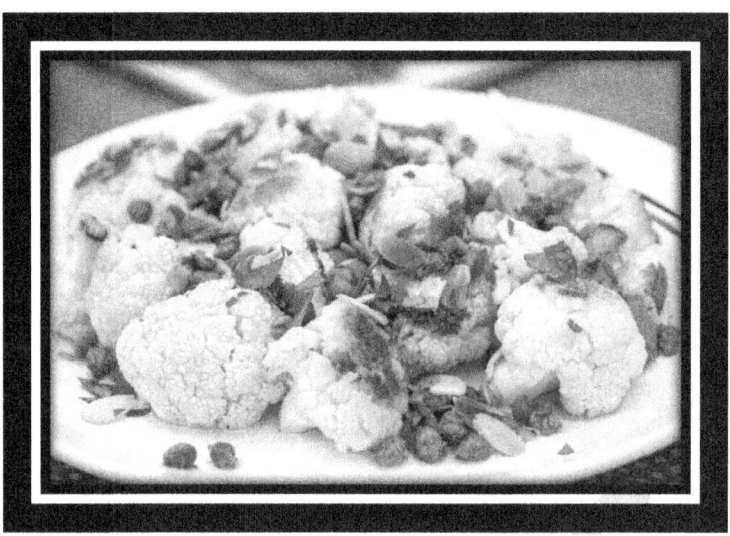

Ingredients:
Servings:4

- 2 tablespoons lemon juice
- ¼ cup extra virgin olive oil
- 2 tablespoons capers
- teaspoon of salt
- 1 tablespoon chopped fresh parsley
- 1 steamed cauliflower

Description:

Whisk together the lemon juice, oil, capers, salt and parsley.
Add cauliflower still warm and cut into small florets and mix well. Serve cauliflower warm or at room temperature in 4 servings.

Nutrition values:
110 calories, 16 gr of fat, 4 gr of carbohydrate, 3 gr of protein

EGGPLANT ROLLATINI

Want to learn how to best cook eggplant? These authentic eggplant rolls may take a little time to prepare, but top end result.

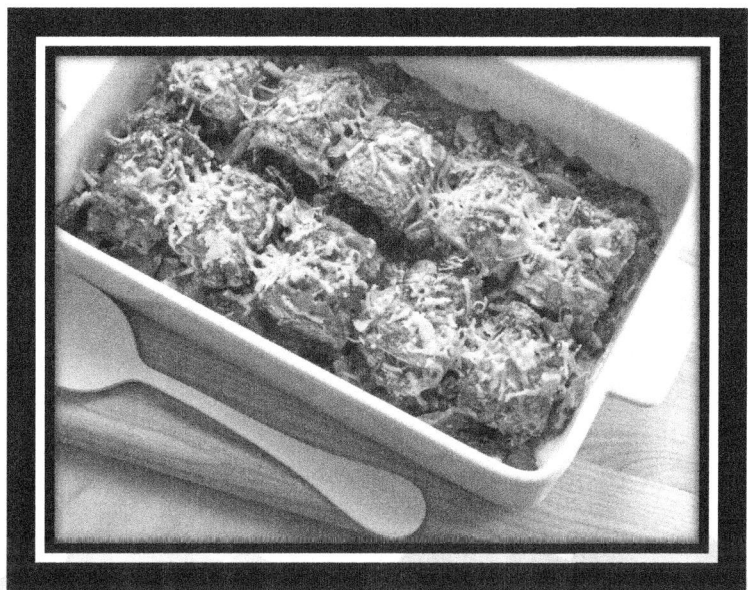

Ingredients:
Servings:4

- ¼ pan of roasted garlic polenta, room temperature
- 2 medium eggplants
- Salt
- Seasoned oil
- 1 roasted red bell pepper
- 2 tablespoons chopped fresh basil
- 2 cups tomato sauce, hot

Description:

Drizzle a glass baking dish with oil and preheat the oven to about 300°.
Cut the polenta into pieces 3 inches long and ¾ inch thick. Cut the eggplant lengthwise into long, ½-inch-thick slices. Remove the skin as much as possible from the first and last slices. Salt the pieces and place them in a colander to drain for 30 minutes. Rinse and pat dry. Brush all eggplant slices with oil and grill until tender.
Arrange a strip of red bell pepper, a sprinkling of basil, and a piece of polenta on the narrow end of the eggplant. Fold the thin end of the eggplant over the polenta and roll up to enclose the filling. Repeat with the remaining eggplant slices.
Spread the tomato sauce in the baking dish. Place the rolls, seam side down, in the sauce.
Bake for 20 minutes until thoroughly browned.

Nutrition values:
325 calories, 18 gr of fat, 36gr of carbohydrate, 36 gr of protein

GREEN BEANS WITH ALMONDS AND MUSTARD

This green bean salad with almonds will delight your palate, and you can enjoy it either warm or at room temperature. Your guests will surely appreciate it.

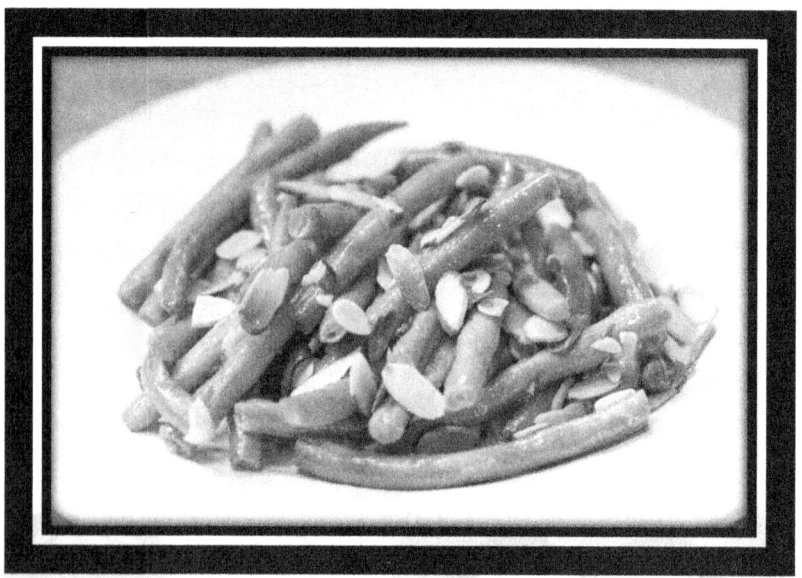

Ingredients:
Servings:4

- 1 pound green beans
- pinch of ground white pepper
- 1/2 cup sliced almonds, toasted
- 1 tablespoon oil
- 1 onion
- ½ teaspoon minced garlic
- ½ teaspoon fresh grated ginger
- 3 tablespoons grainy mustard

- teaspoon sea salt

Description:

Steam or blanch the green beans and keep warm. Heat the oil over medium heat in a large skillet. Add the thinly sliced onion, garlic, and ginger to the skillet and sauté for about 3 minutes or until the onion wilts slightly. Add the mustard, salt, pepper, and 1/2 cup of water to the skillet and bring to a boil. Add green beans and saute until completely coated with sauce. Add half of the almonds and mix well. Pour the green beans onto a serving platter and top with the remaining almonds,and serve.

Nutrition values:
36 calories, 0,6 gr of fat, 7gr of carbohydrate, 1,8 gr of protein

GLAZED TOFU

This is a delicious variation of seared tofu. Adding barbecue sauce if it seems too thick, you can thin it with a little water.

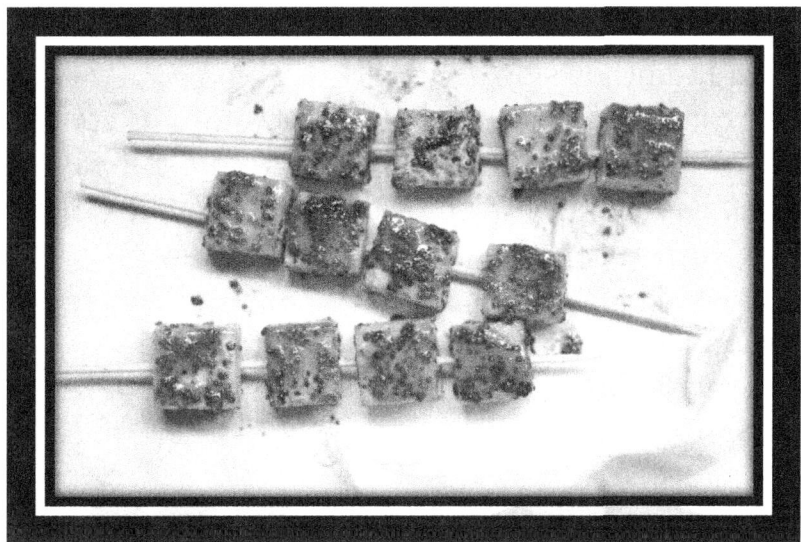

Ingredients:
Servings:4

- 2 teaspoons soy sauce
- 8 ounces of medium tofu
- 1 teaspoon sesame oil
- a pinch of freshly grated ginger
- a teaspoon of minced garlic
- 1 teaspoon sriracha or other hot sauce
- 1 scant teaspoon oil

Description:

Mix the soy sauce, ginger, garlic and hot sauce with 1 teaspoon water in a small bowl.
In a nonstick skillet, heat oil over high heat. Cook tofu for a few minutes (max five min.) until golden brown on one side. For 5 more minutes turn and brown the tofu on the other side...
Add the sauce made earlier. Turn the tofu to coat completely with the sauce. Cook until the pan is dry and the sauce has glazed the tofu. Remove from heat. Drizzle with sesame oil. Serve immediately.

Nutrition values:
108 calories, 0,6 gr of fat, 7,2gr of carbohydrate, 6,3 gr of protein

AFGHAN SPINACH AND TOFU

This spinach afghan recipe will change your perspective towards this vegetable and I'm sure you'll be amazed and left wanting more!

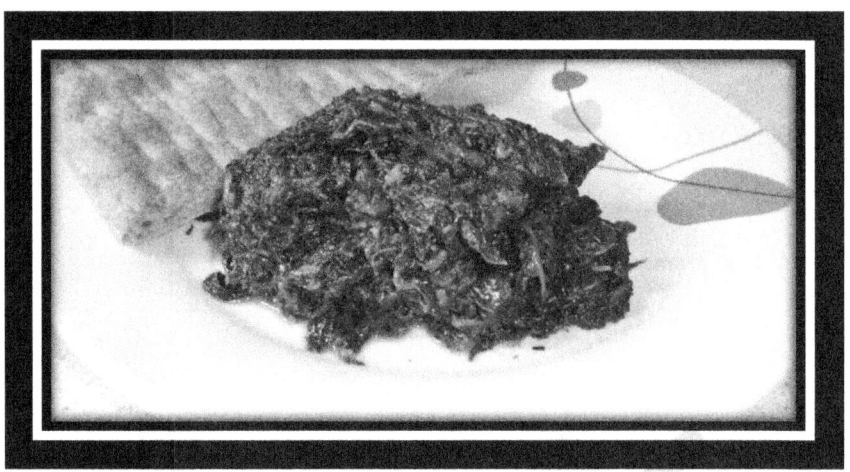

Ingredients:
Servings:4

- Two tablespoons fresh grated ginger
- 2 tablespoons minced garlic
- 2 teaspoons ground cumin
- 2 teaspoons ground coriander
- ½ teaspoon red pepper flakes
- ½ teaspoon ground cinnamon
- 4 cups vegetable stock
- 1 pound silken firm tofu, cut into ¾-inch cubes
- 2 pounds fresh spinach, trimmed and chopped
- 2 tablespoons raisins
- 3 tablespoons oil
- 2 medium onions, cut into ¼-inch slices

- 2 tablespoons soy sauce
- 4 teaspoons sesame oil
- ½ teaspoon sugar
- ¼ cup toasted pine nuts
- Steamed Basmati Rice

Description:

In a crock pot, heat the oil over medium heat. Sauté the onions, ginger, garlic, and spices, stirring constantly. When the mixture becomes fragrant, lower the heat and cook for another 10 minutes. If the mixture sticks, add more oil.

Add the broth to the soup pot and bring to a boil over medium-high heat. Stir to loosen any bits that stick to the bottom of the pot. When the broth boils, lower the heat to medium and add the tofu and simmer for 3 minutes.

Add the spinach and raisins to the soup pot and stir gently. Cover the pot and let the mixture stew for 10 minutes. Add the soy sauce, sesame oil, sugar, and pine nuts and mix well.

Serve over steamed and hot basmati rice.

Nutrition values:
148 calories, 9 gr of fat, 3 gr of carbohydrate, 17 gr of protein

TOFU CURRY IN PUMPKIN

This easy tofu curry, made with beautiful delicata squash and hearty veggies, cooks up in one skillet. The thin skin of the delicata squash is tender when cooked, so there's no need to peel. Serve with quinoa or brown rice.

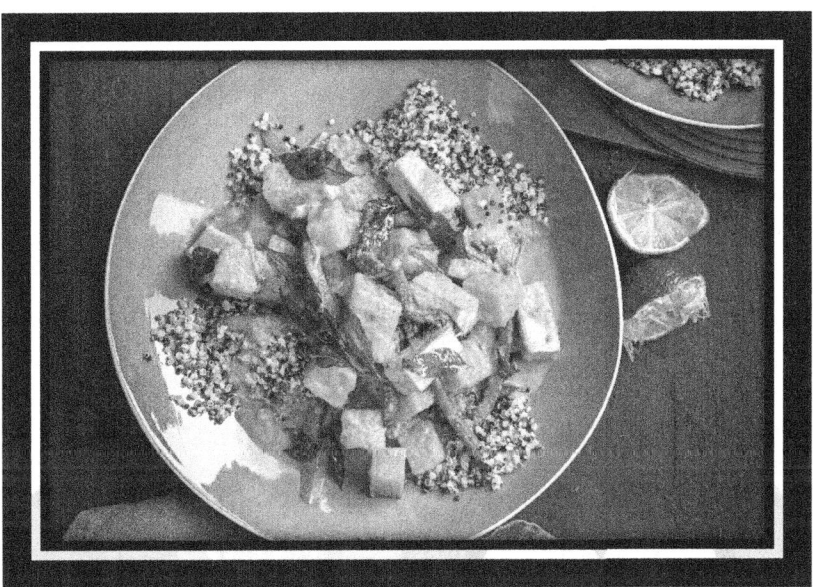

Ingredients:
Servings:4

- 2 small or medium squash
- 1 medium onion, diced
- 2 teaspoons minced garlic
- 2 teaspoons fresh grated ginger
- 2 teaspoons curry powder
- 1 tablespoon oil
- 1 teaspoon ground cumin

- ½ teaspoon ground coriander
- ¼ teaspoon dry mustard
- 1 15-ounce package of solid tofu, cut into half-inch cubes
- 1 red bell pepper
- 1 green bell pepper
- 1 tablespoon chopped basil

Description:

Cut off the stem end of the squash and scoop out the seeds.
Place the squash, cut side down, in a steamer basket over boiling water for about 20 to 30 minutes.
Alternatively, you can microwave the pumpkin faster. Do not overcook the squash, as this will cause it to lose its shape.
Heat the oil in a skillet over medium heat and sauté the onion, garlic, ginger and spices, constantly stirring until the mixture is golden brown. Turn the heat to low and cook for another 10 minutes. If the mixture sticks to the pan, add more oil.
In a small saucepan, simmer the tofu for 3 minutes in 4 cups of water. Gently lift the tofu from the water and add it to the skillet along with the peppers and half of the basil.
Stir gently to mix well—Cook for an additional 3 minutes. Stuff the tofu into the squash and garnish with the remaining basil. Serve with quinoa or brown rice.

Nutrition values:
272 calories, 9 gr of fat, 3 gr of carbohydrate, 16 gr of protein

EDAMAME WITH HIJIKI AND BROWN RICE

Simple and healthy rice dish. Season brown rice with dashi and soy sauce. Then add hijiki and edamame.

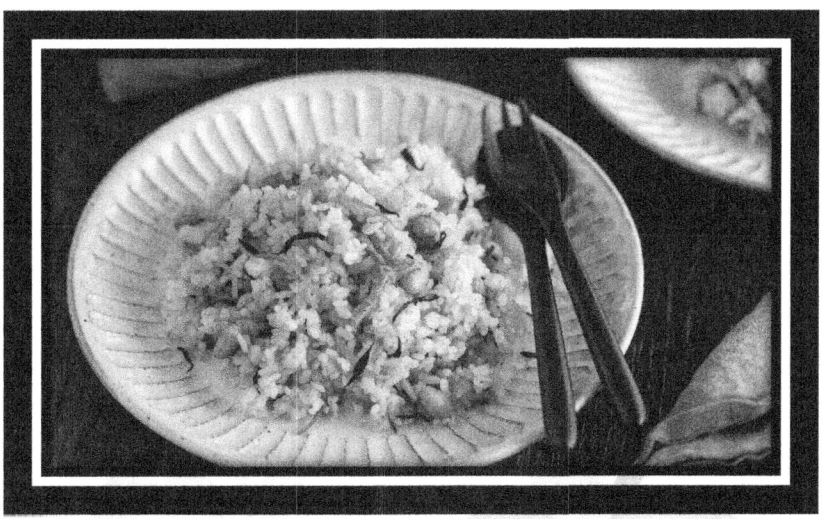

Ingredients:
Servings:4

- ¼ cup hijiki or wakame seaweed
- 1 tablespoon soy sauce
- 2 teaspoons of sesame oil
- 1 tablespoon lemon juice
- 4 green onions, cut diagonally into ¼-inch pieces
- ½ cup shelled edamame, fresh or thawed
- 2 tablespoons canola or grapeseed oil
- 2 cups cooked short-grain brown rice
- ½ teaspoon minced garlic

- 1 teaspoon freshly grated ginger
- 1 medium carrot, cut into matchsticks

Description:

In a small plastic bowl, cover the hijiki with 3 inches of boiling water. Cover and let the seaweed soak for 10 minutes. Drain and set aside.
Whisk with a metal kitchen whisk together the soy sauce, sesame oil, lemon juice and oil in a small bowl. Stir together the rice, garlic, carrot, ginger, green onions, edamame, hijiki,
and the soy sauce mixture. Let stand 20 minutes to allow the flavors to develop. Serve warm or at room temperature.

Nutrition values:
110 calories, 3,5 gr of fat, 8 gr of carbohydrate, 11 gr of protein

TEMPEH IN TOMATO SAUCE

This vegetable-based tomato pasta sauce uses crumbled and ground tempeh to increase the protein content of the dish for a nutritious and satiating evening meal! Serve over steamed basmati rice.

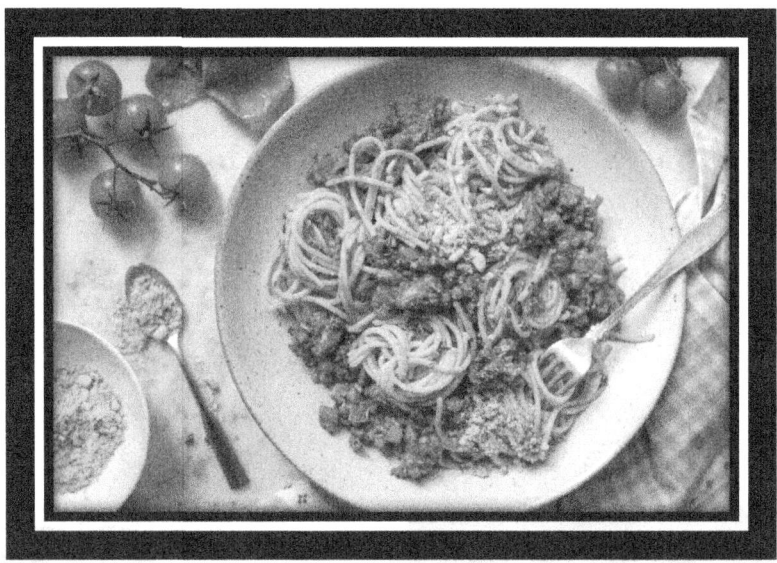

Ingredients:
Servings: 2

- 1 tablespoon oil
- 1 package of tempeh, cut into half-inch thick slices
- Steamed basmati rice
- 2 teaspoons chopped fresh cilantro
- ¼ teaspoon yellow mustard seeds
- 1 onion
- ½ teaspoon chili powder

- ½ teaspoon turmeric powder
- 1 cup diced tomatoes, fresh or canned
- ½ teaspoon salt

Description:

In a large nonstick skillet, heat the oilo over medium heat and add the mustard seeds. When the mustard seeds begin to brown, add the onion, chili powder and turmeric. Cook this mixture for about 15 minutes. Add the tomatoes, salt and tempeh.Cook the resulting mixture for about 10 to 15 minutes until it has thickened and blended well. Serve and accompany with steamed and still hot basmati rice and garnish with fresh cilantro.

Nutrition values:
319 calories, 18 gr of fat, 13 gr of carbohydrate, 34 gr of protein

CONCLUSIONS

However, there are other vegetal foods suitable for the planning of sustainable vegetal nutrition; however, at present, there is no need to avoid soy as a portion of food.

In any case, it is worth the general recommendation to avoid excessive consumption, not because of the unhealthiness of the food, but because nutrition must be varied and therefore, it is necessary to abstain from a diet in which few foods are present with excessive frequencies, causing a monochromatic attitude at the table.

Anyway my advice and suggestion is to always choose one recipe at a time among the many I have prepared and change the type every day for 28 days.

CONDIMENTS AND SAUCE SALADS AND DRESSING

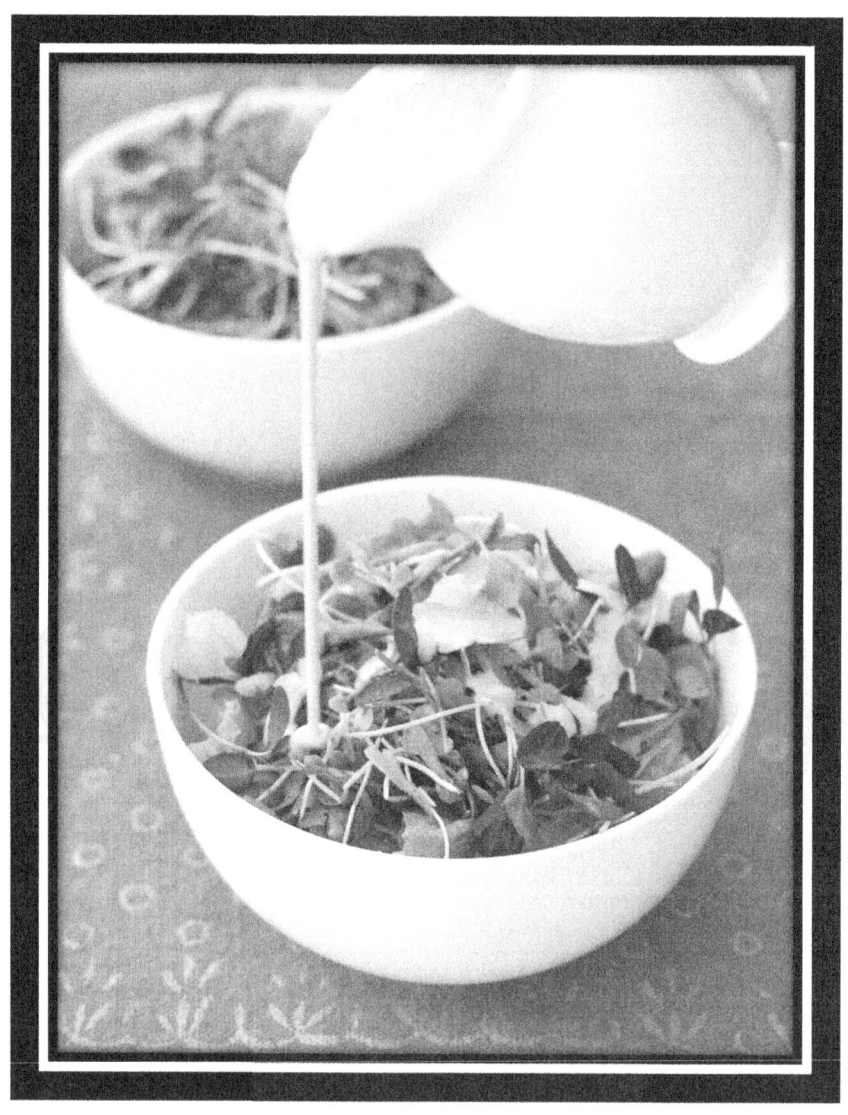

PREVIEW

Many people ignore it, but some of the most libidinous sauces are vegan.

Yes, no animal derivatives, no eggs, and no dairy, simply vegetables, fruits, in some cases a little sugar and oil, but nothing more.

And in the case of recipes like mayonnaise, tartar sauce or hollandaise? Know that making them vegan is a snap.

In short, the universe of vegan sauces is flourishing, and as you know, they can be very useful to enrich appetizers, salads, and sandwiches.

We're ready to take a look at some recipes I've made for you already without dairy, butter or eggs, and others that can be easily transformed, you'll find many recipes on both toppings but especially sauces..

Let's start.

TOFU MAYONNAISE

There are many commercially available soy mayonnaises, but it's easy to make your own at home, not to mention cheaper.

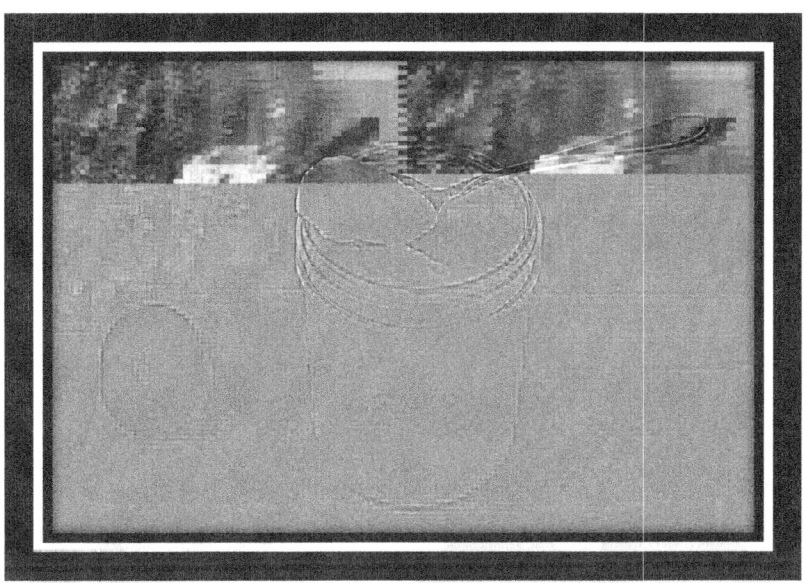

Ingredients:
Servings:6

- 1 pound of tofu
- Two tablespoons fresh lemon juice
- 1 teaspoon Dijon mustard
- 1 tablespoon rice wine or white vinegar
- ¼ cup extra virgin olive oil
- 1 teaspoon white miso or ½ teaspoon salt

Description:

Crumble the tofu thoroughly in the bowl of a food processor or blender. Add remaining ingredients. Process until smooth. Refrigerate for 8-12 hours before using.

Nutrition values:
48 calories, 4,8 gr of fat, 0,1 gr of carbohydrate, 1,2 gr of protein

COOKING KETCHUP

Probably or almost certainly the most famous tomato sauce in the world, ketchup is super versatile and is used in a lot of different recipes to accompany many dishes.

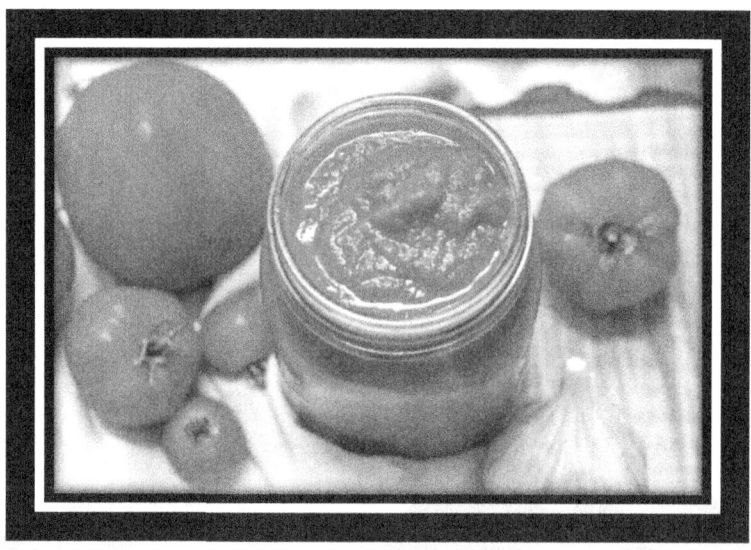

Ingredients:
Servings: 4

- 1 teaspoon oil
- 1 medium onion, diced
- ½ cup apple cider vinegar
- ½ cup sugar
- 1 teaspoon chopped garlic
- 2 teaspoons salt
- a pinch of ground cinnamon
- a pinch of ground allspice
- pinch of cloves

- 1 28-ounce can of diced tomatoes

Description:

In a saucepan or skillet, heat the oil over medium heat. Sauté the onion, garlic, salt, and spices for 8 minutes or until the onion is very soft. Add the rest of the ingredients. Turn the heat high and bring the mixture to a boil. Lower the heat to medium-low and simmer for 15 minutes. Allow the mixture to cool and then reduce it to a puree.
Adjust seasoning with salt, sugar or vinegar and consistency with water.

Nutrition values:
15 calories, 0,8 gr of fat, 4,1 gr of carbohydrate, 0,12 gr of protein

HOT MUSTARD

For a different flavor, try using beer for all or part of the liquid in this recipe. If you want to achieve a yellow color, add ¼ teaspoon turmeric to the mustard powder.

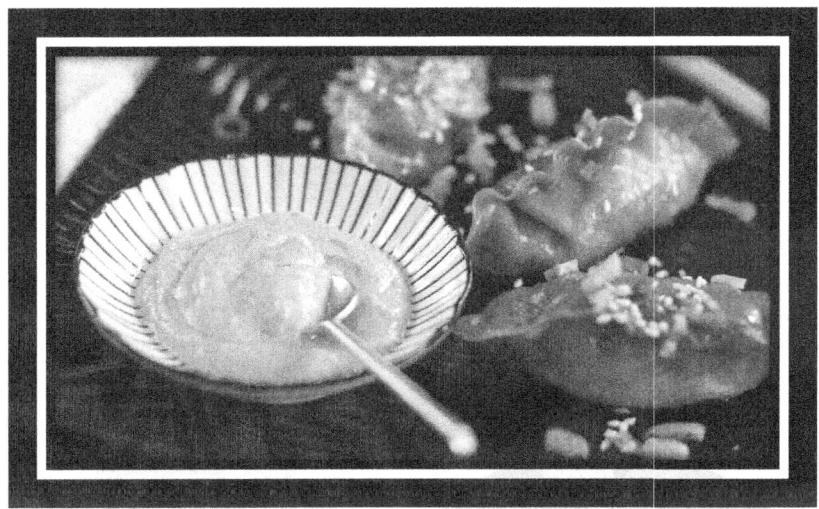

Ingredients:
Servings: 2

- ¼ cup white wine or beer
- ½ cup of dry mustard

Description:

Bring the wine (or beer if you decide to use it) to a boil until reduced by half. Add ½ cup of water. Slowly pour the boiling water into the dry mustard. Allow to steep for about 15 minutes.

Nutrition values:
10 calories, 0,8 gr of fat, 4,4 gr of carbohydrate, 0,12 gr of protein

OLIVE DRESSING

The olive dressing is good for topping Bruschetta or tossed with tomatoes for an impromptu salad. This sauce should be used within 1 week.

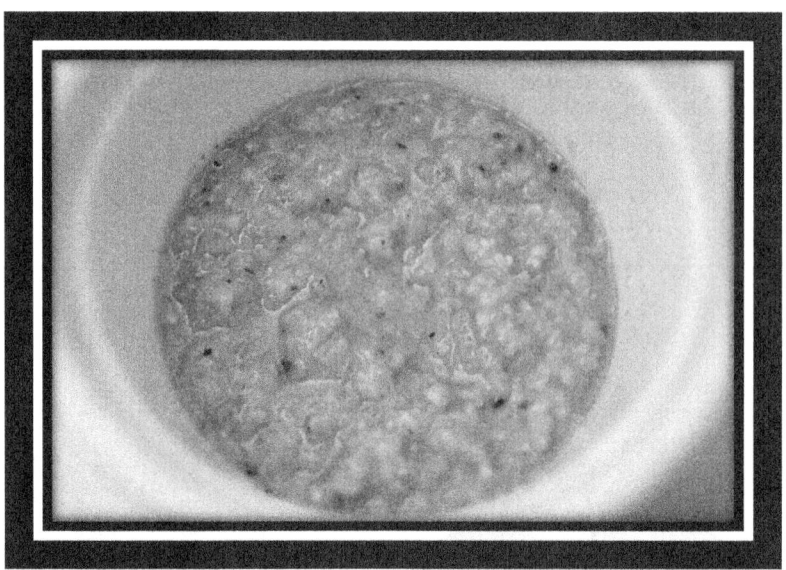

Ingredients:
Servings:4

- 1/2 cup pitted green olives
- 1/2 cup pitted black olives
- 1 tablespoon capers
- cup of chopped roasted red peppers
- ¼ cup diced celery
- 1 tablespoon fresh lemon juice
- 1 teaspoon chopped fresh garlic
- ¼ cup chopped red onion
- ¼ teaspoon black pepper

- ¼ cup red wine vinegar
- ¼ cup extra virgin olive oil
- ½ teaspoon red pepper flakes
- 1 tablespoon chopped fresh basil
- 2 teaspoons fresh chopped parsley
- 1 teaspoon fresh chopped oregano

Description:

Coarsely chop the olives, capers, and red peppers with a sharp knife or chop in a food processor. Combine the olive mixture with the remaining ingredients, taking care to mix well. Let the mixture sit for at least two hours before using.

Nutrition values:
140 calories, 15 gr of fat, 0 gr of carbohydrate, 0,6 gr of protein

GREEN TOMATO SEASONING

This is a quick dressing that takes full advantage of the astringent qualities of green tomatoes.
This sauce will keep in the refrigerator.

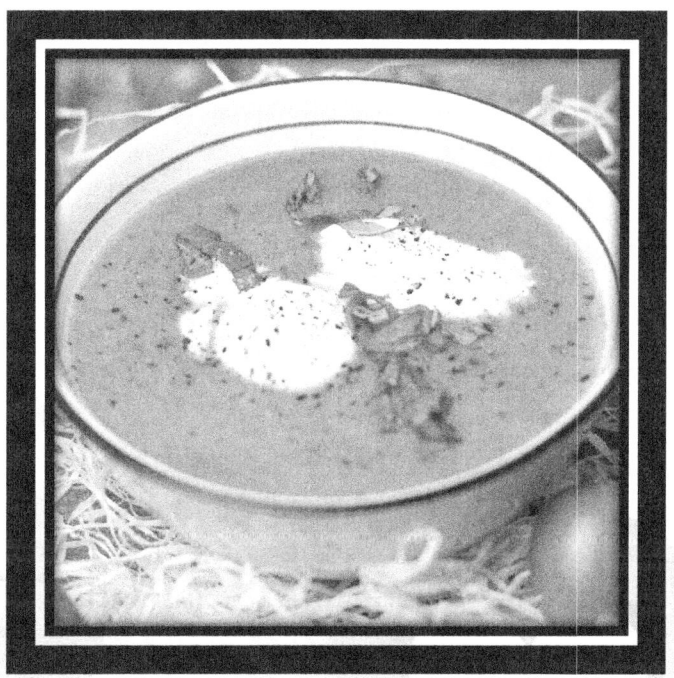

Ingredients:
Servings:6

- Two tablespoons salt
- 1 cup chopped green tomatoes
- 2 medium green peppers, finely diced
- 2 small seedless jalapeños
- 1 medium red bell pepper
- 1 medium yellow bell pepper
- 1 medium yellow onion, finely chopped

- 3 tablespoons brown sugar
- 2 teaspoons mustard seeds
- ½ teaspoon celery seeds
- 1 cup vinegar

Description:

In a large plastic bowl, sprinkle the salt over the vegetables and mix thoroughly.
Let stand for a few hours. Drain the vegetables and rinse them under running water to remove excess salt.
In a large steel saucepan, combine the sugar, mustard seeds, celery seeds, celery and vinegar and bring to a boil for 10 min.
Add the vegetables and bring the mixture to a boil. Place the hot mixture in a glass container with a lid. Once cooled, put the lid on the container, close tightly and refrigerate for several hours before using, even overnight if necessary.

Nutrition values:
41 calories, 15 gr of fat, 0,75 gr of carbohydrate, 6 gr of protein

OKRA PICKLES

For this recipe to be great, okra must be tender, so choose okra the size of your thumb or smaller. If it's more mature, boil the okra with the vinegar and sugar for 5 minutes or until tender.

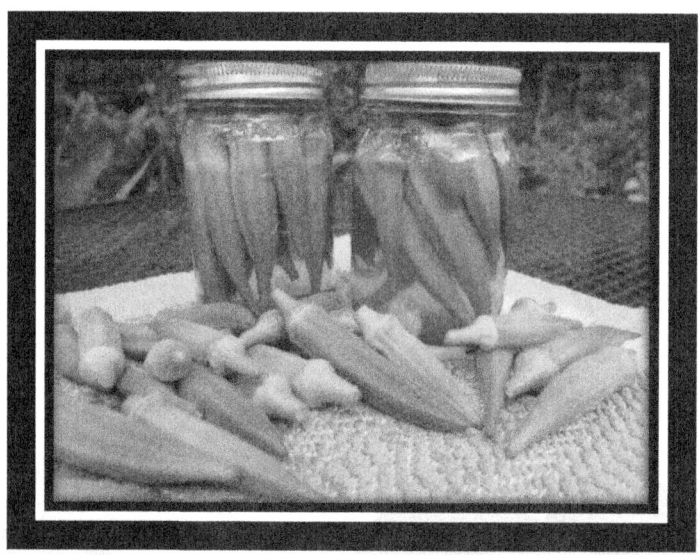

Ingredients:
Servings:4

- 1 red medium onion, cut into long, thin strips
- 1 pound young okra, chopped
- 4 whole cloves
- 6 black peppercorns
- 2 teaspoons mustard seeds
- 1¾ cups apple cider vinegar
- 1 tablespoon salt
- ¾ cup sugar

Description:

Place the onion and okra in a quart jar with an airtight lid.
In a stainless steel saucepan, bring the rest of the ingredients to a boil. Pour over the okra and onions. When the mixture has cooled, place the lid on the jar. When pickles have cooled to room temperature, tighten lid and refrigerate for 8-12 hours before using.

Nutrition values:
15 calories, 0 gr of fat, 12 gr of carbohydrate, 0,2 gr of protein

MUSHROOM PESTO

To make this pesto you can use different qualities of mushrooms to your liking I recommend portobello... Use this pesto to dress pasta or to accompany crostini or bruschetta.

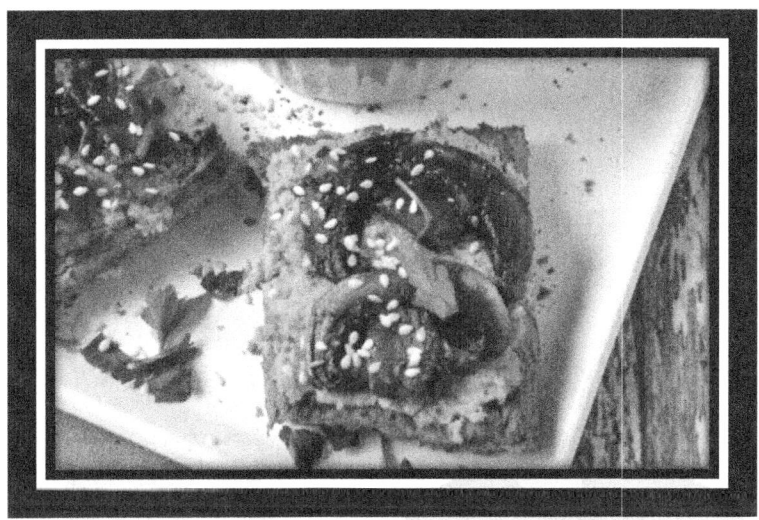

Ingredients:
Servings:4

- 5 medium portobello mushrooms, grilled or roasted
- 2 teaspoons minced garlic
- ¼ teaspoon salt
- teaspoon freshly ground black pepper
- ½ cup walnuts, halved and chopped
- 1 teaspoon fresh rosemary, finely chopped
- ½ cup flat-leaf parsley coarsely chopped
- ½ cup extra virgin olive oil

Description:

Slice the mushrooms thinly and coarsely chop with a knife. In the bowl of a food processor, mix in the garlic, salt and pepper. Let stand for 2 minutes. Add the mushrooms, walnuts, and herbs and process until a thick paste forms. In the processor running, pour the olive oil through the feed tube. Taste and adjust seasonings.
You will get about 2 cups.

Nutrition values:
155 calories, 6 gr of fat, 9 gr of carbohydrate, 7 gr of protein

CONCLUSIONS

Like vegetarians, vegans avoid meat, but they take it a step further and avoid all foods that are animal products, such as milk, eggs and cheese.

To a non-vegan, this may seem limiting, but the truth is that there are solutions for most dishes, including condiments and sauces.

In fact, vegan sauces abound; some, like sauces, have no animal products to begin with, while others, like cream-based sauces, simply swap dairy for something similar to milk but not animal-based.

In general, oil-based sauces are not a problem for a vegan. Salad dressings that incorporate vinegar, tamari or nut butter are fine as long as anything that involves processing animal products, such as some red wines, is left out. Vegan sauces cannot contain butter, but a rich and flavorful substitute can be made with ground sesame seeds.

Have fun and experiment.

DESSERTS AND BEVERAGE

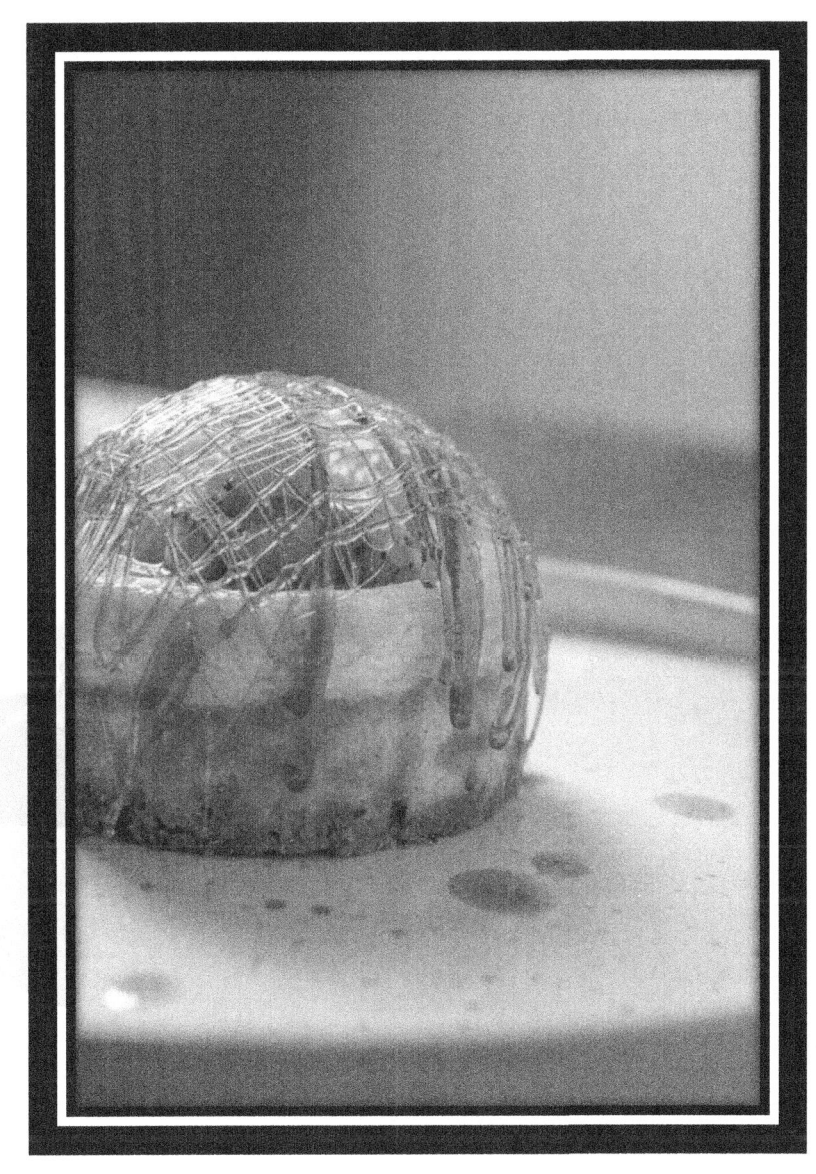

PREVIEW

Arm yourself with spoons and teaspoons because in this collection of recipes, they will be indispensable: I propose to you some of my best vegan spoon desserts, delicious desserts, and drinks to enjoy and serve after lunch or dinner at any time of the year, but also perfect for snacks. To try!

Let's get started.

YELLOW CAKE

You'll love this moist, tender, and fluffy yellow cake made from scratch with delicious white frosting; it's perfect for the holidays.

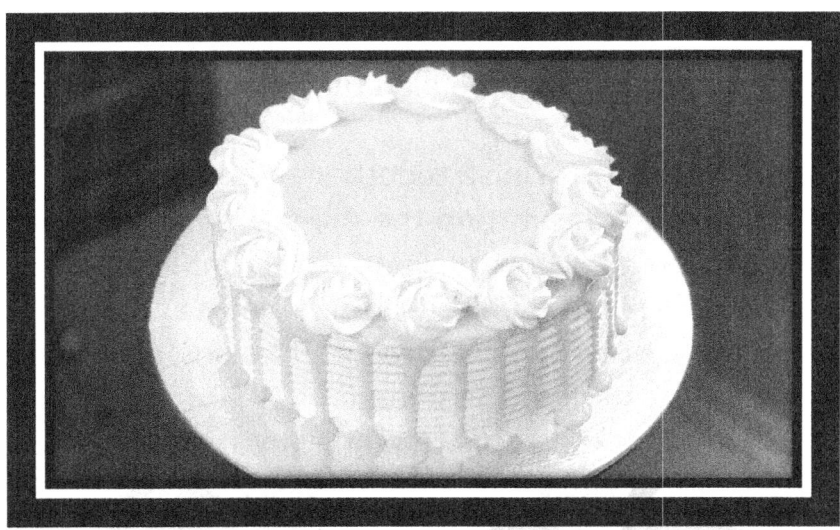

Ingredients:
Servings: 6

- 1½ cups flour
- 1 cup sugar
- 1 teaspoon baking soda
- ½ teaspoon salt
- ½ cup oil
- 1 cup soy milk
- 1 tablespoon vanilla extract
- 1 tablespoon vinegar
- 1 Soft White Frosting Recipe

Description:

Preheat oven to 350°. Cut an 8-inch round out of wax paper.
Lightly grease the bottom of an 8-inch round cake pan. Insert the wax paper onto the bottom of the cake pan. Grease and flour the side and bottom of the cake pan.
In a medium bowl, whisk together the flour, sugar, baking soda, and salt. Add the oil, soy milk and vanilla extract to the flour mixture and whisk until smooth. Add the vinegar to the batter, mix briefly and immediately pour into the prepared baking dish. Bake on the middle rack of the oven for 20-30 minutes or just until the cake begins to pull away from the sides of the pan and the center of the cake looks set. Let cool in the pan for 2 minutes and invert onto a pie plate. Fill and frost with white frosting.

Nutrition values:
355 calories, 15 gr of fat, 49 gr of carbohydrate, 3 gr of protein

THICK CHOCOLATE GANACHE

Chocolate ganache is super easy to make, incredibly versatile, and adds a touch of luxury to anything it embellishes. Spread it on cakes as a chocolate ganache frosting, pour it over sundaes, make fancy drops, or roll it up to make truffles! Any rum or liqueur can be used.

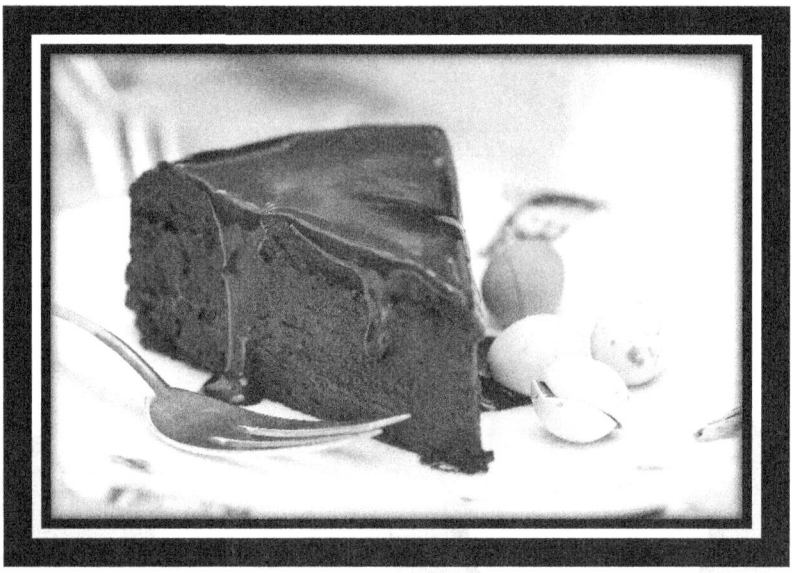

Ingredients:
Servings:4

- ½ cup semi-sweet vegan chocolate chips
- 2 ounces tofu, room temperature
- 1 tablespoon maple syrup
- 1 small dribble of lecithin
- 1 teaspoon vanilla extract
- 2 tablespoons vegan margarine, softened

- 1 tablespoon liqueur or dark rum

Description:

Melt the chocolate chips. Blend the tofu, syrup, lecithin, vanilla extract, and margarine in a blender. Add the melted chocolate while still warm. Allow the ganache to cool in the blender. When the ganache seems quite stiff, add the liqueur or extract and blend until light and fluffy.
It makes enough to generously fill an 8-inch 2-layer cake.

Nutrition values:
362 calories, 13 gr of fat, 36 gr of carbohydrate, 3 gr of protein

LINZER COOKIE SQUARES

These are easy to make and contain less fat than traditional Linzertorten, but have just as much flavor. Most thick jams work for the filling. Make sure the bottom layer of dough seals the pan well.

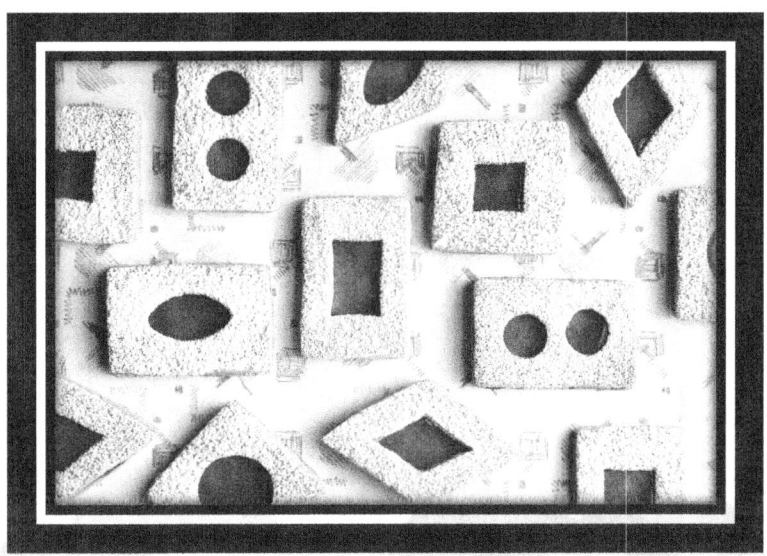

Ingredients:
Servings: 4

- 4 tbsp vegan margarine
- 2 tablespoons oil
- ½ cup corn syrup or barley malt
- 1½ cups flour
- 1 teaspoon vanilla extract
- ¾ cup raspberry jam, preferably seedless
- ½ cup sliced almonds
- ½ cup ground almonds
- 1 tablespoon baking powder

- 1½ teaspoons salt
- ¼ teaspoon ground nutmeg
- ¼ teaspoon ground allspice
- ½ cup water or soy milk
- ½ teaspoon almond extract

Description:

Preheat the oven ventilated to 350° and grease an 11x7-inch baking dish. Beat the margarine, oil, and syrup until light and fluffy. Combine the flour, almonds, baking powder, salt, and spices in a bowl and mix well. Cut the dry ingredients into the margarine mixture until coarse. Add the water or soy milk, the almond extract and vanilla extract and mix until a dough forms.
Taking care that no cracks form, distribute half of the batter into the pan.. Spread the jam over the dough. Crumble the remaining dough into small pieces on top of the jam.
Press the dough together to form a solid layer of dough on top of the jam. Sprinkle the sliced almonds over the dough and press gently into the dough—Bake for 20 to 25 minutes. Wait until the bars are cold before cutting them.

Nutrition values:
211 calories, 5,7 gr of fat, 36,5 gr of carbohydrate, 0 gr of protein

MANGO CREAM PIE

Mango cream pie is a silky dessert made with ripe mango and fresh pastry cream, baked in a shortbread crust.

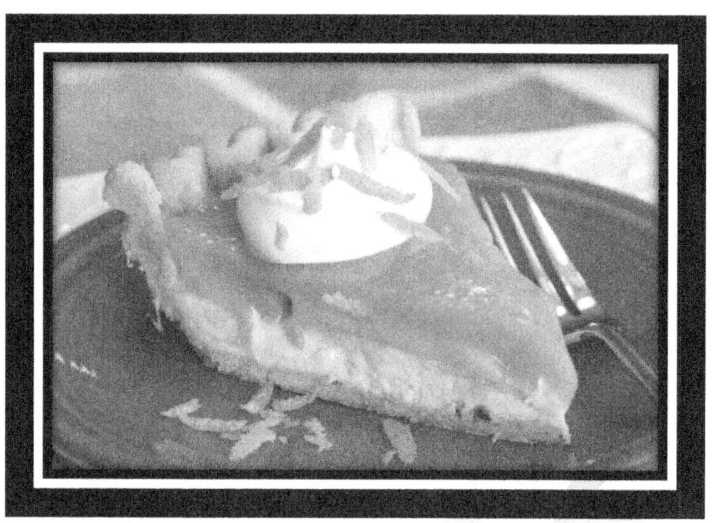

Ingredients:
Servings:4

- 2 teaspoons lime juice
- Tofu cream
- ½ recipe of puff pastry crust
- 1 15-ounce package of solid silken tofu, at room temperature
- 2 large mangoes, peeled, seeded and diced
- 1 teaspoon guar gum
- 1/2 cup sugar

Description:

Roll out the shortbread and bake the tart in a hot oven for 20 minutes.
Blend the tofu with the mangoes. Add the guar gum, sugar and lime juice.
Blend until the mixture is smooth. Pour the filling into the prepared crust.
Cover the pie and refrigerate until well chilled, about 2 hours. Top with the tofu cream.

Nutrition values:
151 calories, 5,7 gr of fat, 3 gr of carbohydrate, 4 gr of protein

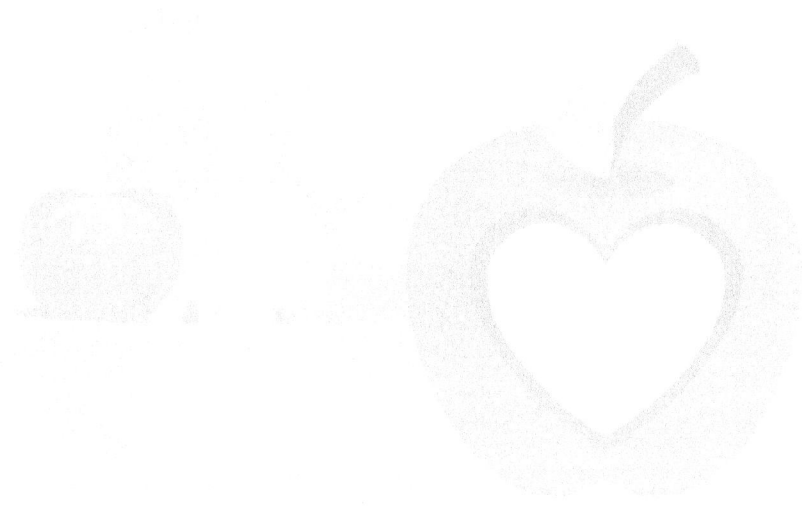

EASY PEACH CRISP

This delicious peach crisp with a generous streusel of ginger and cinnamon is the comfort food of summer.

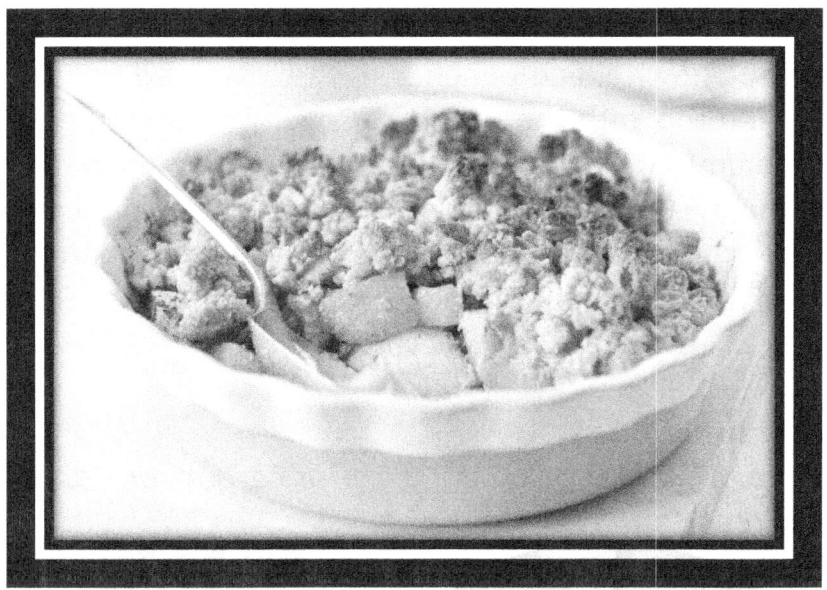

Ingredients:
Servings:6

- 6 cups frozen peaches
- 2 teaspoons lemon juice
- ½ cup sugar
- ¼ teaspoon salt
- ½ teaspoon cinnamon powder
- ¼ teaspoon ground ginger
- teaspoon nutmeg powder
- 1½ cups granola, preferably gingersnap
- 2 tablespoons vegan margarine, melted

Description:

Oil a glass baking dish, preferably 8-inch square and preheat oven to 300° in fan mode.
Mix peaches with lemon juice, sugar, salt and spices in a plastic bowl. Place peaches in the prepared baking dish and top with the granola. Cover the baking dish with aluminum foil and bake until peaches are tender for about 30 minutes. Remove the aluminum foil. Drizzle the granola with margarine. Place the pan under the broiler and gently brown the granola. Serve warm or at room temperature.

Nutrition values:
211 calories, 8,7 gr of fat, 32 gr of carbohydrate, 4,1 gr of protein

SOFT-SERVE ICE CREAM

If you have a ice cream maker, this recipe can be made into a more traditional. The blender method, however, produces a treat for the palate.

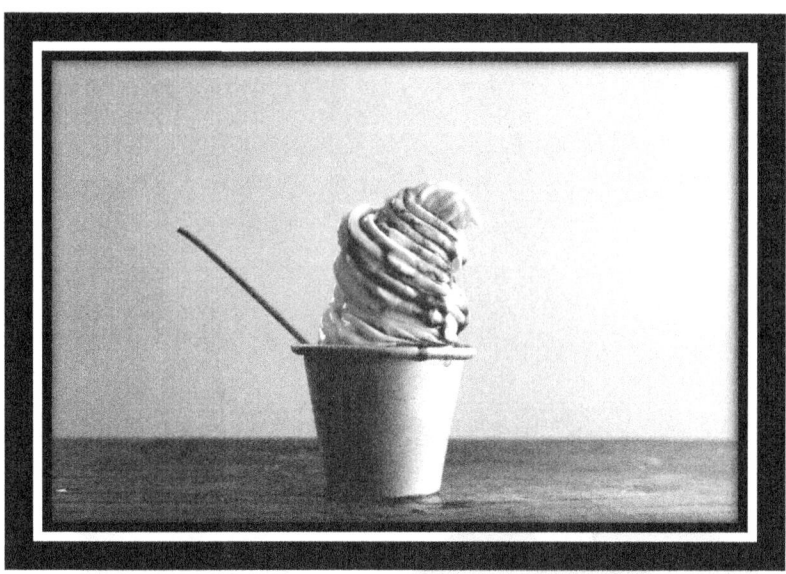

Ingredients:
Servings: 4

- 1 cup flavored soy milk
- 1 10-ounce package of silken tofu
- 2 teaspoons vanilla extract
- Pinch of sea salt

Description:

In a blender or mixer, blend all ingredients until smooth. Freeze the mixture in ice cube trays. When cubes are frozen, grind in food processor until smooth and airy, adding more soy milk if needed. Serve immediately.

Nutrition values:
191 calories, 9,7 gr of fat, 19 gr of carbohydrate, 3,1 gr of protein

BANANA MILK

This is a quick answer to the question, "What do I put on my cereal?
Here's a tasty and easy recipe.

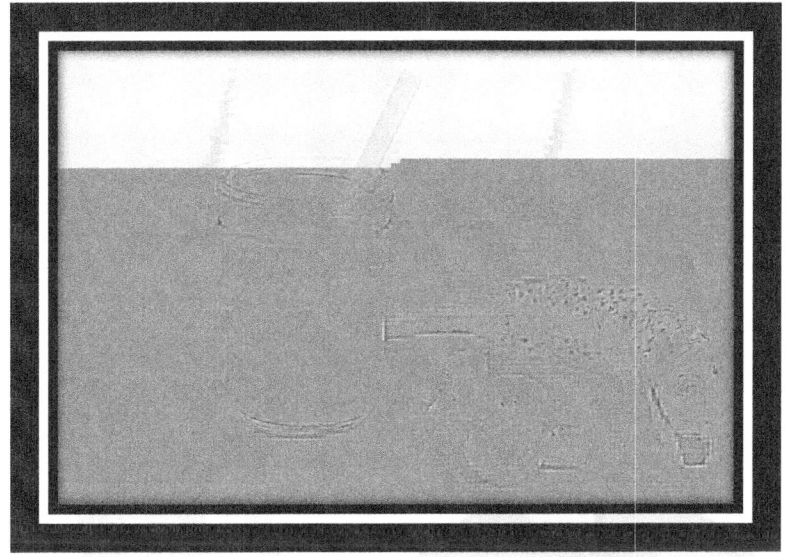

Ingredients:
Servings: 2

- 1 banana
- 1 cup of water
- ½ teaspoon of vanilla extract

Description:

In a food processor or a classic blender pour the banana cut into rounds and then all the other ingredients, blend until you get a smooth and

homogeneous compound. Drink or use immediately, as the banana tends to darken in a short time.
Makes about 1 ½ cups.

Nutrition values:
91 calories, 9,7 gr of fat, 9 gr of carbohydrate, 1 gr of protein

CREAMY ORANGE SMOOTHIE

This creamy, healthy 5-ingredient smoothie tastes like orange Julius and pops combined. Vitamin C has never tasted so good!

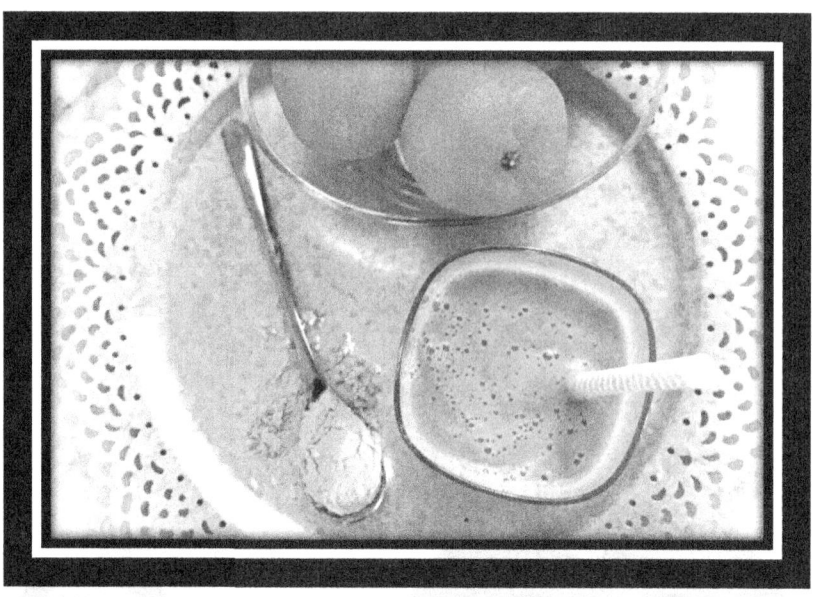

Ingredients:
Servings:4

- 2 cups vanilla soy milk
- 1 16-ounce can of frozen orange juice concentrate
- 1 teaspoon of vanilla extract
- 1 tray of ice cubes

Description:

In a food processor or a classic blender, pour, adding ice last.
Adjust consistency with soy milk, water, juice or ice.
Makes 2 servings.

Nutrition values:
240 calories, 5,7 gr of fat, 39 gr of carbohydrate, 7,1 gr of protein

STRAWBERRY AND BASIL LEMONADE

Strawberry Basil Lemonade. Does this sound a little unusual? It's a little different. When you first take a sip of lemonade you are hit with a sweet strawberry lemonade sensation, then come the bubbles and then the minty fresh basil.

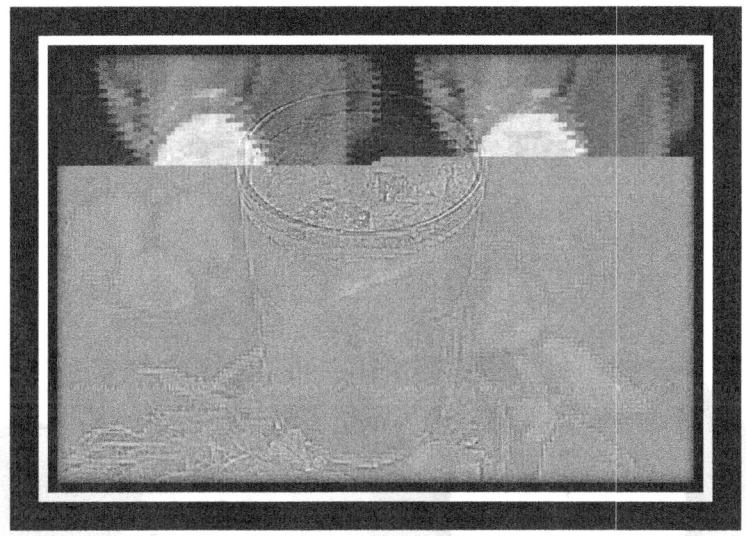

Ingredients:
Servings: 2

- 1¼ cups fresh cut strawberries
- 12 fresh basil leaves
- ½ cup sugar
- 1½ cups fresh lemon juice
- 6 cups water

Description:

In a classic blender, blend the halved strawberries and basil with the sugar. Combine the strawberry mixture, lemon juice and water in a pitcher and mix well. Taste and adjust the sweetness with more sugar. Serve with ice cubes.

Nutrition values:
220 calories, 5 gr of fat, 32 gr of carbohydrate, 3,1 gr of protein

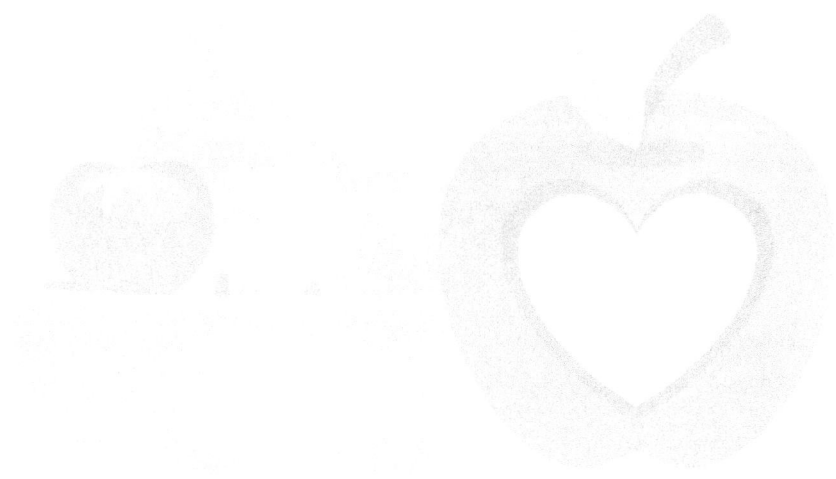

CONCLUSIONS

This chapter on Vegan Desserts and Beverages is also over.

Take a cue from the recipes I have prepared for you, practice, fall in love, and maybe in the future, you will be able to prepare any dish on your own.

FINAL CONCLUSIONS

Approaching vegan cuisine means discovering a wide and colorful variety of foods, dishes, combinations, and recipes, contrary to those who believe that on vegan tables, there are only vegetables and legumes.

Let's try to take a closer look by making what will obviously turn out to be only a partial list as proof of how vast the vegan recipe book is.

Wheat Muscle

One of the most important ingredients of Vegan cooking is certainly Wheat Muscle, very similar to Seitan, rich in proteins, often known as "vegetable meat". Various recipes allow us to prepare it directly at home, while in stores, we will find it in different forms (steak, ham). Wheat Muscle is a product completely of vegetable origin, without saturated fats, rich in essential amino acids, and with about 150 calories for every 100 grams of the product.

Legumes

Legumes and cereals are also absolute protagonists of Vegan cooking. They are typical products of the Mediterranean tradition, but when we talk about cereals, we must always mean the grains of the ears, very rich in fibers, vitamins and minerals, in particular barley, spelled millet, quinoa, wheat and corn. They

are all products very rich in complex carbohydrates, fiber, vitamins, proteins and minerals. Needless to say, the Vegan cookbook includes many dishes made of cereals and legumes, all of them particularly interesting and imaginative.
We can then distinguish whole grains and refined ones; the use of the latter should be pretty moderate. Cooking methods are countless, the only suggestion is to soak them for a period of time varying from six to eight hours; this procedure is necessary in order to avoid phytates remaining inside them, that is the salts of phytic acid present in unrefined grains which prevent our body from absorbing some minerals such as iron, zinc, magnesium and calcium.

Algae

Much less known but of great importance are instead Algae, sources of iodine, iron, calcium, and omega-3 fatty acids. Seaweeds are used to prepare soups, or boiled with oil and lemon; also in this case a suggestion, which is valid for all foods, always avoid exceeding in quantity.

The Vegan diet also includes the use of Dried Fruits, a food which, together with oilseeds, represents an important reserve of minerals, proteins, vitamins and essential fatty acids. The consumption of Dried Fruits should be done regularly, without ever accessing, and preferably walnuts and hazelnuts, pistachios, peanuts, pine nuts. Oilseeds, just as important, turn out to be an excellent alternative to meat and fish, help fight cholesterol and cardiovascular problems and represent an important source of vegetable proteins.

In this field are particularly important pumpkin seeds, sunflower seeds, linseed and sesame seeds, often used for breakfast or as a condiment for legumes and vegetables.

Rice and Soy Milk

For those who cannot give up the consumption of milk, the alternative is represented by rice milk and soy milk; the first one is the Vegan alternative par excellence to cow's milk and does not contain any trace of cholesterol and lactose; the second one is obtained from yellow soybeans and is commercially available both natural and with added vitamins.

Now in this book I have given you many ideas on how to use Vegan Cuisine with the aim of not only losing weight and regaining it, but above all achieving a lifestyle that can improve you as a person both physically and mentally and that you thought was impossible to achieve before. I recommend you to follow the method and the table described here and I am sure that after 28 days you will reach your goal.

Eat, love and live in peace and health.

I embrace you.

Erika Melandri

Printed in Great Britain
by Amazon